was first published in 2003 by
blishing Limited · Phoenix Mill
loucestershire · GL5 2BU

back edition first published in 2005

rary Cataloguing in Publication Data
e recored for this book is available from the British

09 3099 3

10/11.5pt Iowan.
and origination by
lishing Limited.
bound in Great Britain by
& Co. Ltd, Sparkford.

Chloroform

The Quest for Oblivion

To Gary

Chloro

The Quest for

Linda Strat

SUTTON PUBLI

This boo
Sutton P
Stroud ·

This pap

British L
A catalo
Library.

ISBN 0

Typeset
Typesett
Sutton
Printed
J.H. Hay

Contents

J'avais dit, au sujet de l'ether, que c'etait un agent merveilleux et terrible, je dirai du chloroforme, que c'est un agent plus merveilleux et plus terrible encore.

I have said, on the subject of ether, that it is a wonderful and terrible agent, I will say of chloroform that it is still more wonderful and more terrible.

Velpeau and Flourens, 'Communications relatives au chloroforme':
see Chap. 14, n. 51.

PREFACE

When Professor James Simpson, on 10 November 1847, rose to address the gentlemen of the Edinburgh Medico-Chirurgical Society, he was about to realise one of his longest-held ambitions. Some twenty years previously as a young medical student, he had witnessed surgery for the first time. The operation, to remove a breast, was carried out by Robert Liston, one of the leading surgeons of the day. Speed was essential, as was the physical immobilisation of the patient, either by stout leather straps or the hands of burly attendants, since no reliable anaesthetic was then known. The sight and sounds of that operation were a horror that Simpson never forgot. He had fled the theatre in great distress, determined to abandon his cherished study of medicine, and enrol as a law student.

Fortunately he soon thought better of this decision and returned to his medical studies, but he made earnest enquiries of his professors to see if anything could be done to alleviate the terrible pain of surgery. The answer he received was that nothing could be relied upon to relieve the pain with any safety to the patient.

Simpson was not a man to be satisfied with that position, and later, as a qualified doctor, he experimented with a number of methods, including mesmerism. None of them, however, was the thing he sought. While other doctors accepted suffering as inevitable, it was clear that Simpson would not be content until he had found the perfect anaesthetic.

In 1846 news came from America of the development of anaesthesia using ether. Simpson took it up immediately and used it, controversially, in obstetrics, but soon felt that it had too many drawbacks. His use of ether had, however, given him both considerable experience with an inhaled anaesthetic, at a time when many medical men were opposed to its use, and also a standard by which to judge the effects of other volatile chemicals. The quest continued.

On that November day, Simpson prepared with some pride to reveal to the sober gentlemen of the Society his discovery of the anaesthetic powers of a previously little-regarded compound – chloroform. It was common for men of his profession to offer their research and observations for the assistance of their brethren and improvement of the human condition, hoping, also, to gain some personal prestige. All of these must have beckoned, though Simpson was successful enough for the last to be of little import. What he could not have expected was that the events of that November would be the defining moments of the rest of his life. Chloroform would bring him praise and honours, but it would also unleash upon him a storm of outrage. It brought him adulation such as few men ever experience, but when his career moved on to other causes he found that what he had hoped would be his greatest works were little regarded and that, even at the end of his life, all he was remembered for was chloroform. So closely was he associated with it that he was often credited with having discovered it, or administering it to Queen Victoria, neither of which was true.

What he was about to unleash was an agent whose innocuous appearance and pungent but not unpleasant fragrance concealed a dramatic power both to save and to take life. In the years that followed, there would be quarrels, controversy and confusion, with many expressions of pleasure and gratitude, and many deaths. Chloroform would revolutionise battlefield surgery, relieve distressing symptoms in numerous common complaints, and appear to effect astonishing cures – but it would also have a role to play in the crimes of robbery, rape and murder.

At the close of his address, Simpson recommended to the meeting that a committee should be appointed immediately to explore the qualities of chloroform. The gentlemen readily agreed, and the meeting was about to close, but Simpson had a final flourish to perform. He may have anticipated some scepticism, but he knew his audience, and he had come prepared. Never a man to lose the opportunity for drama, he produced a bottle of chloroform and a silk handkerchief, and invited the members to sample its effects. This attitude of almost careless confidence was always to characterise his future use of and total devotion to chloroform. Mr Young, a cutler, at once presented himself as a subject. A teaspoonful of chloroform was applied to the folded fabric, Mr Young inhaled deeply, and after only a few inspirations he was unconscious. A Dr Roberts was the next to try, with the same result. A Mr Hunter followed, and must have taken less than his predecessors, for he suddenly became excited, and jumped to his feet. This caused a certain bustle in the room, as he resisted the efforts of his fellow members to hold him. While this distraction was going on, the handkerchief was being passed around, and one by one the members applied it to their faces. All were surprised by the power of its effect. Gentlemen who might not have arrived at the meeting with the intention of becoming drunk soon found themselves in a state of intoxication. Others, having taken a more concentrated whiff, slumped unconscious in their seats. No doubt Simpson viewed the scene with amusement and satisfaction. Once recovered, the doctors were agreed that the sensation was delightful, and some were eager to repeat the experiment. Fortunately, no one was the worse for his experience. Had one of the audience died on that occasion, as might very well have happened, the future of chloroform would have been in some doubt, and history would have been a little bit different.

A NOTE ON MEDICAL STATUS

In nineteenth-century Britain only those medical men who were members of the Royal College of Physicians were entitled to call themselves 'Doctor'. It is not always possible in contemporary material to identify the status of individuals, so for the sake of clarity, I have referred to all qualified medical practitioners as 'Dr' unless they had another title such as Professor, or a military rank.

ACKNOWLEDGEMENTS

I would like to extend my grateful thanks to the following individuals and organisations whose assistance in the preparation of this book has been beyond value: the Association of Anaesthetists of Great Britain and Ireland; Bellevue Hospital Archives, New York; the British Library; Cuxson Gerrard and Co. Ltd; Edinburgh City Archives; the Family Record Centre; the History of Anaesthesia Society; the Jefferson County Historical Society; the London Metropolitan Archives; the National Museum of Health and Medicine, Washington; the Newspaper Library, Colindale; the Nuffield Department of Anaesthesia, Oxford; the Royal College of Physicians, London; the Royal College of Physicians, Edinburgh; the Royal College of Surgeons, Edinburgh; the Simpson House, Edinburgh; the Society of Authors; the University of Edinburgh Archives.

A special mention is due to three people who have been extraordinarily generous with their time in steering me through the minefield that is the medical and chemical literature of chloroform – they are Dr Ray Defalque, Dr Harry Payne and Professor James Payne.

I owe a particular debt of thanks to Jaqueline Mitchell, for her unfailingly helpful and always excellent advice.

The encouragement and faith of one's friends should never be underestimated. Gail, John, Liz – take a bow.

Finally, a big thank-you is due to my husband Gary, who, as well as giving practical help and support, has shown tremendous patience and fortitude in spending so many months living with a woman whose sole topic of conversation appeared to be chloroform.

ONE

Give Me to Drink Mandragora

> The escape from pain in surgical operations is a chimera, which it is idle to follow up today. 'Knife' and 'pain' in surgery are words which are always inseparable in the minds of patients, and this necessary association must be conceded.
>
> *Velpeau, a leading surgeon of his day, writing in 1839*[1]

In 1847 chloroform blazed on to the Victorian scene like a comet, whose muted beginnings were forgotten in scenes of brilliant light and grim shadow. Some regarded it with horror and despair, others predicted its rapid passing, but for many it was a triumph of science over nature, and the harbinger of a bold new age of medicine. To the confident and optimistic, chloroform appeared to be the ideal, the perfect anaesthetic that had been sought by humankind since the dawn of time. This heady excitement was soon to evaporate, but for many years to come, chloroform was widely used, abused and misused in human society.

To understand the reaction of the Victorian medical profession and public to the appearance of chloroform, we must first take a short tour of the history of anaesthesia, which is at least as long as recorded history itself. However, while there is ample information on the subject, it is hard to judge the effectiveness of early attempts at pain relief during surgery since the degree of success reported tends to depend on whether the writer is a surgeon, an academic, or a patient.

From earliest times, the possibility of anaesthesia has thoroughly engaged the minds of commentators on the human physical condition. Early *Homo sapiens* must surely have noticed that intense pain or a blow on the head would sometimes lead to unconsciousness, a state that mimics natural sleep but during which the patient (or, maybe, the victim) feels no pain. This observation would have stimulated the desire, and later the search, for some artificial means of procuring a pain-free slumber.

Possibly the first depiction of painless surgery in literature is in the Bible, when God causes Adam to fall into a deep sleep while He removes the rib from which He makes Eve. After the couple's fall from grace, God issued a decree, the precise meaning of which is still a matter for lively debate. Henceforth, Adam must toil to bring forth food from the ground, while to Eve God said, 'I will greatly multiply thy sorrow and thy conception; in sorrow thou shalt bring forth children.'[2] The Bible therefore appears to associate painless surgery with the brief period of humankind's innocence, and the travail of childbirth with the decline into sin, a distinction which was not lost on some nineteenth-century obstetricians.

EARLY PAIN RELIEF

The earliest attempts at pain relief probably used soporifics such as opium and alcohol, both of which have been available far longer than written records. Alcohol on its own was known to numb the senses, though its effects were short-lived, especially as pain could lead to rapid sobering of the patient. However, it was often used to carry doses of other drugs.

The unripe seed heads of the opium poppy yield a milky juice rich in alkaloids, of which the most important is morphine. The juice could be dried for storage and later mixed with water and alcohol. Its sedative and sleep-inducing properties made opium a valued aid to medicine, but it had two major drawbacks: it was poisonous; and it was addictive. It was not, of course, an anaesthetic, but for someone about to undergo surgery it was very much better than nothing. Despite the availability of soporifics, however, 'nothing' was what the patient often received. This meant that if a surgeon was to be able to operate effectively, the only thing to do was to tie or hold the patient down and work quickly.

Although the Greeks and Romans knew about opium, their writings make little mention of pain relief. It is not clear, therefore, whether the second-century Greek physician Galen, who advised opium and mandragora for the relief of pain before performing operations, was typical of his time or an enlightened exception. The Greek essayist and biographer Plutarch, describing a first-century operation on the Roman general Caius Marius for tumours in his legs, did not refer to any methods of alleviating pain – rather he praised the patient for his fortitude. Marius elected not to be tied down, but having endured the cutting of one leg without flinching or making a sound, he declined to allow the surgeon to touch the other, commenting, 'I see the cure is not worth the pain'.[3] Celsus, a Roman encyclopaedist writing about surgical practice in AD 30, advised that the ideal surgeon should be among other things 'so far void of pity that while he wishes only to cure his patient yet is not moved by his cries to go too fast or cut less than is necessary'.[4]

Another plant with a long history of use for medicinal and social purposes is *Cannabis indica*, which grows naturally in Asia and India and produces a resin that has been used from early times to ease pain, induce sleep and soothe nervous disorders. In AD 220 the Chinese physician Hua T'o was said to have performed extremely complex surgical procedures without causing pain after administering a preparation of cannabis in alcohol. Unfortunately, his patients have left no record of their experiences.

Mandragora officinarum, a native of southern Europe whose root and bark have long been known to have soporific properties, is related to the deadly nightshade. It was described in *Historia Naturalis*, a 37-volume work written in about AD 77 by Pliny the Elder that included the medicinal use of herbs among its many subjects and retained its influence throughout the Middle Ages. According to Pliny, mandragora was 'given for injuries inflicted by serpents and before incisions or punctures are made in the body, in order to insure insensibility to pain. Indeed for this last purpose, for some persons the odour is quite sufficient to induce sleep.'[5] This may be the first recorded reference to pain relief during surgery being produced by inhalation.

The Greek pharmacologist Dioscorides, who lived in the first century AD, prepared the first systematic pharmacopoeia, *De Materia Medica*. It was translated and preserved by the Arabs, and finally translated back into Latin by the tenth century. This suggested that the root of the mandragora plant be steeped in wine and given 'before operations with the knife or actual cautery that they may not be felt'.[6] Mandragora had its dangers, however, which may have led to some caution in its use. Aetius, a Greek physician writing at the end of the fifth century, remarked on the effects of an overdose of mandragora, stating that a patient given too much would gasp for breath, became convulsed, and, if assistance was not given, die. This description has the ring of personal observation.

Mandragora continued to be used with caution for many hundreds of years. Bartholomeus Anglicus, who compiled an encyclopaedia of natural history in 1235, stated: 'the rind thereof medled with wine . . . gene to them to drink that shall be cut in their body, for they shall slepe and not fele the sore knitting'.[7] The thirteenth-century Spanish chemist, Arnold of Villanova, gave the following recipe:

> To produce sleep so profound that the patient may be cut and will feel nothing as though he were dead, take of opium, mandragora bark and henbane root equal parts, pound them together and mix with water. When you want to sew or cut a man dip a rag in this and put it to his forehead and nostrils. He will soon sleep so deep that you may do what you will. To wake him up, dip the rag in strong vinegar.[8]

A contemporary surgeon, Hugo of Lucca, refined this method. He added the juice of lettuce, ivy, mulberry, sorrel and hemlock to the above and boiled it with a new sponge. This was dried and when wanted dipped in hot water and applied to the patient's nostrils.

The properties of mandragora were still well known in the early seventeenth century. Shakespeare mentioned it in *Antony and Cleopatra*, when the Egyptian Queen demands:

> Give me to drink mandragora! . . .
> That I might sleep out this great gap of time
> My Antony is away.[9]

Hyoscyamus niger, commonly known as henbane, is found throughout central and southern Europe, western Asia and India, and was well known by the first century AD for its action in pain relief and inducing sleep. The main constituents are the alkaloid hyoscyamine with small amounts of hyoscine and atropine. The plant was recommended by Dioscorides, though Pliny declared it to be 'of the nature of wine and therefore offensive to the understanding'.[10]

It is also mentioned in medical works of the tenth and eleventh centuries, and by Elizabethan herbalists such as

Nicholas Culpepper, an apothecary who in 1652 wrote his famous herbal *The English Physician*, and John Gerard, who in 1597 published his *Historie of Plants*, a compendium of the properties and folklore of plants.

Later it seems to have fallen into disuse, and is omitted from eighteenth-century pharmacopoeias. Gerard wrote that the juice caused 'an unquiet sleep, like unto the sleep of drunkenness, which continueth long and is deadly to the patient',[11] and Culpepper advised that it should never be taken internally at all. In the Middle Ages the fumes obtained from heating the seeds were a popular treatment for toothache, though it was observed that there was considerable risk in its use, as its actions were uncertain and could lead to dangerous side-effects.

THE ABANDONMENT OF OLD KNOWLEDGE

The works of Galen, the Arab physician Avicenna, and the Greek 'father of medicine' Hippocrates were the basis of medical knowledge until the Middle Ages. Universities studied the old texts but added nothing to them. Since medieval philosophers held that the forms of nature were determined by God, it was not felt necessary to explain how things worked. Medicine was based on superstition, folk remedies, herbs, astrology and prayer.

While there were no real advances in pain relief up to the mid-nineteenth century, one might imagine that the old tried and tested herbal soporifics would continue to be employed in the absence of something better. The evidence of those who actually experienced or observed surgery tells a different and remarkable tale. Surgery after the Middle Ages was a terrifying and bloody agony, and the early methods of pain relief were largely abandoned.

Why did this happen? Some historians admit that they don't know the answer. Others skate so carefully around the gap that one has to look carefully to find it. Still others say, in the face of considerable evidence to the contrary, that since the old soporifics were available they 'must' have been given. A few offer explanations, that there was a Renaissance backlash against the practices of the ancients, that opium, henbane and mandragora were not as effective as had been claimed and were dangerous in use, or that medical and religious tracts suggested that pain was in some way essential to the proceedings. All of these suggestions have some element of truth.

In the fifteenth century, improved translations of the classic texts created a renewed interest in Greek and Roman medicine, and this eventually spawned a counter-movement, whose most influential voice was the Swiss physician who called himself Paracelsus. He certainly believed in sweeping away the old beliefs, for in 1527 he publicly burned the revered works of Avicenna and Galen in front of the University of Basel. He believed in personal observation rather than books, and, importantly, he ushered in the study of the chemistry of the body and medicine. After his death his followers continued his work and, ignored by the universities, obtained private funding for their laboratories. Science and religion were still linked, and God was still the creator, but man could use science to explain the nature of the universe.

The movement gained ground, fuelled by advances in scientific method and inventions such as the microscope. The works of Galen and Hippocrates were no longer regarded with unquestioning veneration, and their remedies could be tested. While the old drugs were still used, it was no longer claimed that they produced anaesthesia, and it was realised that complete pain relief was only possible at great risk to the patient.

Nineteenth-century surgeons were extremely sceptical of the efficacy of such measures as Hugo of Lucca's anaesthetic sponge. Dr John Snow, the leading London anaesthetist of his day, examined the prescription and announced his utter disbelief that such a sponge as prepared would, after being placed in hot water, give off any odour or vapour that would cause insensibility. He thought that if sleep were really caused by it, some of the moisture on the sponge might have reached the mouth or throat and been swallowed, his reason being that that the main ingredient was hemlock, which is not volatile enough for inhalation.

Snow also referred to a description written by Theodoric, the son and student of Hugo of Lucca, of patients about to undergo an operation being tied down or held by strong men. In operations for hernia Hugo directed that the patient be tied to a bench or table with three bands; one round the ankles, one round the thighs and one across the chest holding down the arms and hands. This hardly suggests a confidence in the anaesthetic.[12]

Henry J. Bigelow, professor of surgery at Harvard University, declared in 1876 that the essentials of a modern anaesthetic were that insensibility should be always attainable, complete, and safe. By contrast, he described stupefaction with poppy, henbane, mandragora and hemp, as partial, occasional and dangerous.[13] Certainly, prior to the development of instruments for the sensitive measurement of drugs and the establishment of dosages, the amount of active principle in a herbal preparation must have varied enormously, with highly unpredictable results.

It is tempting to conclude with the nineteenth-century doctors that if their predecessors had had, as they claimed, a safe and successful method of preventing pain, it would not have fallen into disuse. The patient might well have felt that some pain relief was much better than none at all, but many doctors were chary of using strong soporifics, and while there were a few who were willing to make their patients drunk to the point of stupor before an operation, this practice was generally condemned.

A great deal of progress would be needed before anaesthesia could become possible, particularly in the development of the science of chemistry and the evolution of sensitive measuring apparatus. Meanwhile, just as doctors unable to prevent infection assumed that suppuration was normal and desirable, and welcomed the appearance of 'laudable pus', so they also declared that pain was a necessary and beneficial part of surgery, and deplored attempts to relieve it as not merely wrong, but dangerous. Medically, pain was a stimulant – it was good for you – while morally it was a punishment for sin, or a test of faith for the holy. If this was true of surgical pain, it was doubly true of the pain of childbirth, which was a perfectly natural thing with which it was unnecessary to interfere.

SURGERY AND PAIN

Descriptions and illustrations of surgery in the seventeenth to mid-nineteenth centuries are mainly a catalogue of unrelieved agonies. An account of an amputation by John Woodall of St Bartholomew's Hospital, written in 1639,[14] makes no mention of pain relief, but refers to the surgeon requiring five helpers, two of whom were to assist the surgeon with his instruments and needles, and the other three to restrain the patient. It was normal practice to locate the operating theatre of a hospital as far as possible from the main wards, often in a tower room, so the shrieks of the unfortunate patient could not be heard by those destined to suffer the same fate.

Despite Celsus's recommendation that a surgeon be without pity, it is clear that many felt acute distress at the sufferings they were about to inflict. William Chesleden, one of the most distinguished surgeons of his day, was said to have suffered great mental anguish on operating days. His method of sparing the patient agony was speed, and he was able to complete a lithotomy (extraction of stones from the bladder) in less than one minute. In 1731 he recommended a draught of opium for the pain, but that was after the operation, not before. John Hennen, a deputy inspector of military hospitals, suggested in 1820 that 'many of the primary operations would be rendered much more favourable in their results by the administration of a single glass of wine',[15] which does rather suggest that in some cases the patient was not even receiving that much.

A few doctors were eager to experiment with various means of reducing pain during surgery. Quite apart from humanitarian considerations, there was a great advantage to the surgeon. The cries and struggles of the unfortunate patient were distracting and distressing. The surgeon was obliged to hurry to complete his work and had little or no time to consult with colleagues when difficulties were encountered. Muscle spasms made treatment of fractures and dislocations especially difficult, and many delicate or lengthy operations, while technically possible, could not be performed on a conscious patient.

Some of the methods tried sound drastic and even dangerous. Many would only have been suitable for certain operations and robust patients. In the sixteenth century the effect of the tourniquet in dulling pain was well known, and was occasionally used in cases of amputation. An English surgeon, James Moore, suggested in 1784 that compression of the nerve trunks should be practised before cutting the area supplied by them, and John Hunter carried out this method for the amputation of a leg at St George's hospital. A French surgeon, Richerand, declared that a dislocated hip was easily corrected after a bottle of port wine, though the main object of intoxication was muscular relaxation rather than pain relief. The seventeenth-century Italian physician, Marco Aurelio Severino, used a mixture of snow and ice to numb the skin before operations, applying it in narrow parallel lines for only fifteen minutes to avoid tissue death. Other methods used were compression of the carotid arteries to produce unconsciousness, and encasing the head in a helmet to which a sound blow was delivered with a wooden hammer! Philip Syng Physick of Philadelphia, referred to as 'the father of American surgery' decreased sensitivity to pain by bleeding patients to a state of collapse. In the 1790s he reported an operation in which after the bloodletting he was able to manipulate a dislocated joint. The patient, he stated, was entirely relaxed and seemed to feel no pain.[16]

One method that was extremely successful, with no risk at all to the patient, was hypnosis. This met with all the enthusiasm that one might have expected of the nineteenth-century medical establishment. The first accredited operation under hypnosis, a mastectomy, took place in France in 1829, but the authorities denounced the patient as a fraud and the doctor as a dupe. A Scottish surgeon, Dr James Esdaile, practised most of his working life in India, and there performed his first operations under hypnosis in 1845. Despite thousands of painless operations to his credit, on such conditions as piles, scrotal tumours, and compound fractures, with the mortality rate an amazingly low 5 per cent, the British medical profession refused to take his work seriously. John Snow was quite unable to believe in hypnosis. He thought that Esdaile and other surgeons had been 'imposed upon by dishonest and designing patients, who afterwards confessed they *had* suffered the pain to which they had pretended to be insensible'.[17] Alternatively, he suggested that the patients were susceptible persons in whom a condition resembling hysteria or catalepsy had been produced.

In the early nineteenth century, therefore, patients were still being tied or held to the operating table, fortified only by the power of prayer, though not a few might have had a stiff 'bracer' before the event. A patient undergoing lithotomy in 1811 at St Thomas's Hospital in London described his experience:

> My habit and constitution being good, it required little preparation of body, and my mind was made up. When all parties had arrived I retired to my room for a minute, bent my knee in silent adoration and submission and returning to the surgeons, conducted them to the apartment in which preparations had been made. The bandages etc., having been

> adjusted I was prepared to receive a shock of pain of extreme violence and so much had I over-rated it, that the first incision did not even make me wince although I had declared that it was not my intention to restrain such impulse, convinced that such effort to restrain could only lead to additional exhaustion. At subsequent moments, therefore I did cry out under the pain, but was allowed to have gone through the operation with great firmness . . . and when the words, 'Now Sir, it is all over' struck my ear, the ejaculation of 'Thank God, Thank God!' was uttered with a fervency and fullness of heart which can only be conceived. I am quite unable to describe my sensations at the moment. There was a feeling of release, not from the pain of the operation, for that was gone and lost sight of, but from my enemy and tormentor with a lightness and buoyancy of spirits, elating my imagination to the belief that I was restored to perfect health as if by a miracle.[18]

That more complex surgery was done without pain relief can be illustrated in the letter written by Professor George Wilson to James Young Simpson, blessing him for inventing chloroform anaesthesia. In 1843, Wilson had a Syme amputation of the foot, which involves a disarticulation of the foot with preservation of the heel pad. After the removal of the foot, the heel pad is swung forward as a flap, and attached to the stump. Once healed it will eventually bear weight. Wilson wrote:

> Of the agony it occasions, I will say nothing. Suffering so great as I underwent cannot be expressed in words, and thus fortunately cannot be recalled. The particular pangs are now forgotten, but the black whirlwind of emotion, the horror of great darkness, and the sense of desertion by God and man, bordering close to despair, which swept through my mind and overwhelmed my heart, I can never forget however gladly I would do so.[19]

THE BEGINNINGS OF INHALATION ANAESTHESIA

Henry Hill Hickman, born in Shropshire in 1800, was probably the first person to attempt anaesthesia using an inhaled gas. A member of the Royal College of Surgeons from 1820, he conducted a number of well-documented experiments on small animals in 1824. When he placed a puppy under a glass dome filled simply with air, he saw that the animal gradually became unconscious, and he was then able to surgically remove one of its ears without it showing any signs of pain. The animal survived, and in later operations lost the other ear and its tail. Hickman went on to use carbon dioxide to produce unconsciousness in animals, and removed the leg of a dog, the ears of a rabbit and the ears and tail of a kitten. He published the results of these experiments in an open letter dated 1824 but it was given little attention. In 1826 the *Lancet* published a derisive letter headed 'Surgical Humbug' from someone signing himself 'Antiquack', in which Hickman's letter was denounced as 'a decoy by which the credulous may be induced to give up their senses as well as their cash', and his procedures, which were effectively the production of asphyxia, were condemned as 'occasioning sensations far more horrible than the pain inflicted by ordinary operations'.[20] Hickman went to Paris in 1828 and asked for permission to perform his experiments there, but nothing came of this and he returned to England where, dispirited, he died in 1830.

Help, however, was at hand for suffering humanity. It had been at hand but unrecognised for centuries. It is not known for certain who first demonstrated the action of sulphuric acid on alcohol to produce what was known as 'sweet oil of vitriol'. This may have occurred as early as the thirteenth century. The colourless volatile liquid, light enough to float smoothly on water, was highly inflammable and potentially explosive. The vapour had a distinctive penetrating odour, and a tendency to make people cough. In 1540, Valerius Cordus, a German botanist and apothecary, described its preparation, but it was Paracelsus who observed the hypnotic effect of the liquid after mixing it with the feed of chickens, recording that after a long sleep they awoke unharmed. More than 300 years were to pass before another scientist noted the effect. In 1730, the German chemist W.G. Frobenius renamed it 'ether'. Its mode of preparation led to its later appearance in the literature as 'sulphuric ether'.

The eighteenth century saw a renaissance of chemical and medical research. Doctors still had very little idea of what caused diseases, and most of their remedies were little more than palliatives, if they worked at all. However, as new compounds emerged from chemists' laboratories and new elements were identified, the hope arose that among these modern marvels might be that elusive thing – a 'cure'. The only way for doctors to find this cure was to try out any likely looking substance, on animals, on patients, and on themselves. In 1758, Dr Michael Morris explained the method of preparing ether to the Society of Physicians in London and related three cases in which he had 'cured' lumbago and rheumatism by rubbing it on the affected parts. The cold caused by the evaporation of the ether had created local anaesthesia.

In 1775, Joseph Priestly, already noted for his work on electricity, published a six-volume series called *Experiments and Observations on Different Kinds of Air*. Not only had he been one of the first to isolate oxygen, but he had also discovered nitrous oxide, a colourless gas with a slightly sweet aroma. Medical men were very excited about the new gases, and were eager to experiment by inhaling them, as well as the vapour of volatile liquids, to see if they had any therapeutic effect, especially for respiratory diseases.

In the 1790s English physicians Richard Pearson and Thomas Beddoes started using ether in the treatment of asthma, consumption, catarrhal fever (influenza), bladder stones, and scurvy. As a bronchodilator it may have relieved some respiratory symptoms. In 1798 Beddoes founded the Pneumatic Institution for Inhalation Gas Therapy in Bristol, then a thriving centre for patients coming to enjoy the mineral waters. His object was to combine a laboratory for the investigation of therapeutic gases with a small hospital. His advertisements offered permanent cures for consumption, paralysis, and venereal diseases, and while orthodox doctors denounced him as a quack, patients flocked for his free treatments. The gases they inhaled were mixed with air and included oxygen, carbon dioxide, nitrogen, and even carbon monoxide, which was thought to improve health as it gave the patient pink cheeks! Beddoes's assistants were destined to outshine their master, for he employed Humphry (later Sir Humphry) Davy and the engineer James Watt to help manufacture the gases. As might be expected, the treatments offered no real benefit, and eventually even Beddoes ceased to believe in them. Patients did not return, even when offered money as an inducement, many of them feeling they were being experimented upon. When Davy left in 1801 the work dwindled to nothing and the Institution was closed in 1802. It was Davy who coined the term 'laughing gas' after inhaling nitrous oxide and discovering its pleasurably intoxicating effects. He noticed, however, that it also had the property of destroying physical pain and in 1800 observed 'it may probably be used to advantage during surgical operations in which no great effusion of blood takes place'.[21]

It was more than forty years before anyone followed up this observation, and in the meantime 'nitrous oxide capers', where the public would pay to inhale the gas, became a feature of travelling carnivals. It created a dreamy, floating, drunken sensation, but also made the participants giddy so that they staggered about and became objects of amusement to onlookers.

In 1818 an article on the subject of ether appeared in the *Quarterly Journal of Science and Arts*.[22] The authorship is unknown, but it is popularly attributed to Michael Faraday, then working as an assistant to Humphry Davy, and three years away from his more famous work on electromagnetism. He pointed out the resemblance between the effects of ether vapour and those of nitrous oxide gas but advised caution, since following an experiment with ether, a man had remained in a lethargic state for more than thirty hours and there had been fears for his life. This warning prevented serious investigation for a number of years. In the 1820s and 1830s, American physicians confirmed Faraday's finding that ether and nitrous oxide were similar in effect, but this was seen more as a laboratory curiosity than something capable of practical application. The careful use of ether continued. In 1833 a Dr James Hurd was treating a patient with an abscess by inhalation of ether diluted in hot water. She became exhilarated, hummed tunes, and lapsed into unconsciousness for half an hour. He was so terrified he determined never to try it again.[23] When ether and nitrous oxide were eventually recognised as anaesthetics this would emerge not from the laboratory, but from their recreational use.

Public interest in the sciences in the nineteenth century had led to the popularity of lectures by travelling 'professors' at which members of the audience would be invited to inhale the new intoxicants. Afterwards, medical students would retire to their lodgings and continue the experiments, not always with a scientific purpose in mind, and as the public heard about this so the practice spread. The custom of 'ether frolics' was duly added to the nitrous oxide capers. Since fluid ether was more easily transported than a bag of gas, it was now possible to have an ether party in your very own home. From time to time, a participant would be obliged to sleep off the effects, but several years were to pass before anyone thought this was an interesting development.

In 1839, William Clarke, a medical student of Rochester, New York, began entertaining his friends with ether inhalations. On an unknown date, possibly as early as January 1842, Clarke administered ether on a towel to a Miss Hobbie who then had a tooth painlessly extracted by her dentist, Elijah Pope. Clarke's failure to publish an account of this groundbreaking event suggests that he didn't fully appreciate its importance.[24]

In 1841, Dr Crawford Long of Jefferson, Georgia, introduced the practice of inhaling nitrous oxide to the young men of the town, and later changed to using ether. A mischievous soul, he used the excuse of mild intoxication to get away with kissing all the girls at parties. The fashion soon spread to other parts of the state, where reeling students could sometimes be seen inhaling ether in the street or on campus. Long had often discovered when recovering from the effects of ether that there were bruises on his body which he could not recall suffering, and wondered if operations could be performed painlessly under its influence. The first recorded use of ether as a surgical anaesthetic occurred on 30 March 1842, when Long used it in the removal of two tumours from the neck of James M. Venable, who felt no pain from the procedure and paid two dollars for his treatment. Long went on to perform other minor operations using ether anaesthesia, but although his methods were known in his immediate neighbourhood he refrained from publishing the results. His lack of any sense of urgency seems astounding, and his chief apologist was his wife, who pointed out that older doctors in the area were sceptical of the practice and Long felt he needed more time to perfect it, a difficult task in a small town where surgery was infrequent. He was also under the impression that the real answer to anaesthesia would come from current work on hypnosis. He finally published an account of his work in 1849 in the *Southern Medical and Surgical Journal*, but by then two major developments had taken place.

The first serious promoter of nitrous oxide anaesthesia was a dentist from Hartford, Connecticut, Horace Wells. Wells had inhaled nitrous oxide during a stage demonstration by a Dr

Gardner Quincy Colton, who after receiving his degree had chosen a career of lectures and demonstrations. On 10 December 1844 he gave a gas demonstration at Hartford, which was attended by Wells. One of the audience, a young man named Sam Cooley, danced about the stage under the influence of the gas and ran against some wooden settees, injuring his knees without noticing the pain. Wells, who was shortly due to have a molar extracted, at once saw the relevance of this to dentistry. He persuaded Colton to bring a bag of gas to his surgery the next day. Colton brought it along in a rubber bag fitted with a tube and administered the gas to Wells, the tooth being extracted by his associate, Dr Riggs. Wells, who had felt only a little discomfort, was very optimistic. After some further experiments, he was confident of the value of this discovery. Convinced that he would make his name, he arranged a demonstration before a group of medical students in January 1845 at the Massachusetts General Hospital. It was a failure, for by mistake the gas bag was with-drawn too soon and the patient (who later claimed he had felt far less pain than usual) was only partly anaesthetised, and groaned loudly during the operation. An unruly audience cried 'Humbug!', Wells was humiliated, and he left Boston. His continued attempts to promote nitrous oxide failed. In 1847 the Paris Medical Society looked favourably on his work, but when he returned to the United States, it was to find ether established and chloroform the new rage. In January 1848, he spent a week repeatedly testing chloroform to the point of addiction and under its influence rushed out into the street and threw acid over the clothing of two women. He was committed to the Tombs Prison, his life in ruins. There, he committed suicide by inhaling chloroform to the point of analgesia, then slitting an artery in his leg with a razor. He was thirty-three.

In 1846, a one-time partner of Wells's dentistry practice, William Thomas Green Morton, asked his former tutor Charles T. Jackson about the production of nitrous oxide gas. In the previous two years, Jackson had been experimenting with ether. He had realised that earlier difficulties were due to impurities, and had succeeded in purifying it so it could be inhaled without danger. He had intended to develop it for surgical purposes, but lacking the time to do the work himself, he responded to Morton's enquiry about nitrous oxide by recommending ether as having a similar effect. Morton began to experiment with ether, and that year painlessly extracted a tooth from Eben H. Frost, who was asked to sign a statement to say that he had felt no pain. H.J. Bigelow was invited to observe a number of extractions and, as a result, a demonstration of ether anaesthesia took place at the Massachusetts General Hospital on 16 October 1846. Morton administered the ether, but the surgery, to remove a tumour from the neck of twenty-year-old Edward Gilbert Abbott, was carried out by a leading surgeon, Dr John Warren, the patient afterwards claiming not to have felt any pain. 'Gentlemen,' Dr Warren remarked to the enthralled audience, 'this is no humbug.'[25]

In November 1846, Oliver Wendell Holmes, an eminent physician and father of the future Supreme Court Justice, wrote to Morton suggesting that the state produced by the agent be named anaesthesia, from the Greek *an* for 'without' and *aesthesia* for 'sensibility'. The word was not previously unknown, but Holmes's suggestion led to its common use.

Morton, certain that ether would make his fortune, refused to disclose the nature of the solution, added a few harmless impurities to try and disguise the smell, named it 'Letheon' (in Greek mythology, the waters of the River Lethe were held to expunge painful memories), and persuaded Jackson to join him in taking out a patent. They distributed circulars to doctors demanding half the fee in the case of any operation in which it was used. Dr Bigelow was not to be fooled. He soon discovered by its characteristic smell that Letheon was ether and sent the news to his friend Dr Boott of London. The day after receiving the news, Dr Boott tried the administration of ether in his own house at Gower Street while a neighbouring dentist, James Robinson, removed some teeth from a patient without causing any pain. This operation performed on 19 December 1846 was the first in which ether vapour was employed in England as an anaesthetic.

Morton's attempts to capitalise on the process led to his being discredited. When Jackson tried to claim that he was the originator of the discovery, the partnership and the friendship came to an abrupt end. Morton spent the rest of his life neglecting his business and spending his money trying to obtain recognition, and ultimately became bankrupt. When he was forty-nine, in the July heat of New York in 1868, his mind finally gave way. Trying to drive out of the city in his buggy, he reached

Central Park, then suddenly stopped, leaped out and collapsed, probably from a stroke. He died later in hospital.

Jackson spent many years attacking Morton's claims to have originated the use of ether. Embittered, he turned to alcohol. Five years after Morton's death he was found, raving drunkenly, at Morton's graveside, where the stone commemorated his rival's contribution to anaesthesia. He spent the remaining seven years of his life in an asylum, dying at the age of seventy-five.

With nitrous oxide temporarily disgraced, ether was the sensation of the day, although not everyone embraced the new concept of anaesthesia. The differences between the conscious and unconscious states were little understood, and the effect of anaesthetics on the brain was a mystery. Sleep was believed to be a halfway house between consciousness and death, during which the brain, apart from maintaining basic functions, was inactive. The higher functions of the brain, the essence of what made an individual human, were therefore locked in the state of consciousness, and to remove these was to reduce man to little more than an animal. The creation of artificial unconsciousness therefore raised the spectres of madness and idiocy. It was not only life, reason and intellect that were at risk, for the search was still in progress for the physical seat of the human soul, which might be in some part of the nervous system as yet not fully understood. Dr James Parke of Liverpool stated:

> I contend that we violate the boundaries of a most noble profession when, in our capacity as medical men, we urge or seduce our fellow creatures for the sake of avoiding pain alone – pain unconnected with danger – to pass into a state of existence the *secrets* of which we know so little at present. . . . What right have we even as men, to say to our brother man 'sacrifice thy manhood – let go thy hold upon that noble capacity of thought and reason with which thy God hath endowed thee . . .'[26]

Numerous contributions to the medical and general press show that, in the main, the detracting voices were few and surgeons welcomed the use of ether, although it did have its drawbacks. The smell was both unpleasant and persistent, and it irritated the airways, while large amounts were required for protracted surgery. It was slow to take effect, creating an initial state of violent excitement undesirable in delicate operations. In February 1847 it was reported that in a recent experiment, a man under the influence of ether had suddenly sprung up, jumped over three chairs and attacked an onlooker.[27] It had taken six men to restrain him. Ether's easy inflammablity was very worrying in the days of open fires, gas jets and candlelight. (Mr Young, the cutler who had been so keen to be Simpson's guinea-pig, had once offered himself as a volunteer in a test where he was rendered unconscious with ether while a flame was held to his mouth. He survived.)[28] What was needed was an anaesthetic that was simple to administer, requiring only small quantities, yet giving a rapid and complete effect, nonflammable for preference, and with a pleasant smell into the bargain. The answer was chloroform.

TWO

SWEET WHISKEY

I presume it was little suspected that such things were doing in a remote region on the shore of Lake Ontario.

Professor Benjamin Silliman[1]

In 1872 the eminent German chemist Justus von Liebig published a paper claiming the honour of being the original discoverer of chloroform.[2] His only rival to that title, he believed, was the leading French pharmacist Eugène Soubeiran, who was in no position to argue the point, having died in 1858. The true discoverer of chloroform, however, was an industrious and eccentric amateur, the American Dr Samuel Guthrie. These three men produced chloroform independently and within a few months of each other, each by a different method. None of them knew what he had made.

Samuel Guthrie was born in Brimfield, Massachusetts, in 1782. His father, also Dr Samuel Guthrie, was a practising physician and surgeon of Scottish descent. Young Samuel studied medicine with his father and began his own practice in Smyrna County, New York. In 1804 he married sixteen-year-old Sibyl Sexton, and they started raising a family. In the war of 1812 Guthrie was an examining surgeon and took part in the second battle of Sackets Harbor. After the war he returned to medical practice but before long had set his sights on another career, starting what was to be a lifetime of manufacturing ventures, independent research and experiment.

In 1817 Guthrie was looking for a piece of land on which he could start a commercial enterprise, and recalled the pleasant location of Sackets Harbor on the shores of Lake Ontario. About a mile east of the harbour was a tract of land, almost a wilderness, but with considerable potential. It was good farming country, near a thriving port, and most importantly there was Mill Creek, a source of water power. Guthrie purchased the land, and with his wife and three children set off to make a new life. The area eventually became known as Jewettsville, after Abram Jewett, another 1817 arrival, who set up a brickyard. In the following years, industry flourished, and the village soon boasted sawmills, lime kilns, coopers' shops, blacksmiths, a rope factory and three vinegar mills.

Guthrie was a resourceful man of great energy and ingenuity. He believed in wasting nothing. Soon he had cleared the land, built a home from local materials, piped water from a nearby stream, and planted his first crops, walling the area with the stones he had excavated from the soil. Until his commercial ventures matured he continued to practise as a doctor, and also articulated skeletons, which he sold to medical schools. Visitors and servants were sometimes horrified when opening containers in the house to discover them full of human bones. He was regarded with some awe by his neighbours and was considered a little peculiar by medical colleagues. A slender, stooping figure, with a prominent nose and expressive eyes, he had a thoughtful demeanour, and in common with so many great thinkers, dressed plainly and was a little careless of his appearance. He abhorred extravagance, but never grudged spending on scientific experiment.

By 1820 Guthrie's tremendous industry had established him as a formidable presence in the neighbourhood. He had built a substantial brick house, which still stands today, barns and outbuildings for his farm, a distillery, vinegar factory, gunpowder mill, workshop and chemical laboratory. In his library were to be found works on medicine and chemistry, as well as scientific journals. The products of his businesses supplied Madison Barracks, a local military post, or were shipped to New York for sale. He also cultivated forty acres, planted a vineyard and raised cattle, sheep, poultry and hogs. This would seem to leave no time for recreation, but he enjoyed hunting and fishing, and the occasional game of whist, and sometimes entertained his family and friends on the violin. He was not, however, a man for idle conversation, and much of the time he was to be found in his laboratory or workshops, where he was occupied in a lifelong fascination with explosives.

Disappointed by the slowness of ordinary gunpowder he determined to devise an improved priming powder. It was extraordinarily dangerous work. Every so often the villagers would hear a muffled explosion and see Dr Guthrie running out of his powder mill with eyebrows singed and face and arms scorched. He once claimed in a letter to have had about 100 explosions from the percussion powder alone, some of them very severe, the largest amount he had burned at one time being 30 pounds.[3] On one occasion he had received the blast from a quarter of a pound of powder full in his face and eyes. In the middle of writing that letter he recorded that he had been obliged to break off and rush out of the house, because of a loud noise and a shrill scream of 'Fire!' from his alcohol distillery. The history of his accidents, he said, would fill a volume. The worst one was from putting his hand into a keg containing four pounds of percussion powder and cracking a piece of it between thumb and finger. The friction set fire to the powder and the resulting detonation resulted in terrible burns to his hand and arm, and tore most of the skin from his chest, neck and face. He was lucky not to lose his arm. His grandson described another such incident that lifted the roof off the workshop and flattened the walls; only the fact that the door opened outwards saved the occupants from injury. Altogether Guthrie was involved in eleven major explosions, and was often seriously burned, twice nearly fatally. Sometimes he was so badly burned that he did not want to be seen, even by his family, until some healing had taken place. While he recovered, a bed would be made up for him in the laboratory and meals would be passed to him through the slightly open door. Despite these incidents, which did permanent damage to his health, he did not give up this work until he was satisfied with the product, which was eight and a half times faster than common gunpowder. He also compounded the powder into small pellets, which achieved a wide sale.

Such was the success of his business ventures that Guthrie, even though there were now four children to provide for, was able to abandon the medical profession and spend more time on his experiments. In 1830 his sons, Alfred and Edwin, were old enough to take over many of the business activities, and in the next two years, before they left to pursue their own careers, Guthrie devoted a great deal of his time to his laboratory. The results of his work were published in the *American Journal of Science*, whose founder and editor, the noted pioneering chemist and geologist Professor Benjamin Silliman of Yale College, would receive boxes packed with small bottles of the compounds produced by Guthrie. One such project, which Guthrie undertook in 1830, was an attempt to produce sugar from potatoes. He didn't succeed, but did make what he called 'potato molasses', which was glucose syrup.

Early in 1831, Guthrie read an entry in Silliman's *Elements of Chemistry*[4] that greatly interested him. Silliman described how in 1796 an association of four Dutch chemists who had already discovered the gas ethylene (C_2H_4), which they called 'olefiant gas', studied the effects of mingling it with chlorine. Chlorine (Cl_2) had been discovered in 1774 by the Swedish chemist Carl Wilhelm Scheele, but it was not until 1809 that it was recognised as an element. Its compounds were widely used for bleaching and fumigation.

The result of the Dutch chemists' experiment was a dense oily-looking liquid with an interesting ethereal odour and a sweet taste, which they called 'chloric ether', though it was popularly known as 'Dutch liquid'. They had not been able to discover its composition, and for many years it was a little-regarded curiosity. Silliman had been in the habit of preparing an alcoholic solution of the liquid in his laboratory at Yale, sipping it diluted with water and calling the attention of the medical students to its 'remarkably grateful properties as a cordial',[5] suggesting that it might prove to be invaluable in medicine. By 1831 it was known to be a compound of carbon, hydrogen and chlorine ($C_2H_4Cl_2$), and though its medical potential had not been explored, Silliman declared it was highly probable it that would be an 'active diffusive stimulant'.[6] This liquid we now know as ethylene dichloride. It is inflammable and highly irritant when inhaled. It is mainly used in the manufacture of PVC and as a pesticide, and is not considered suitable for human consumption.

The Dutch chemists' method of producing their liquid resulted in only a small yield of the promising product from a large volume of gas. Guthrie scented commercial potential, and at once started experimenting to see if he could produce the liquid in a simpler and cheaper way. He decided to start by combining, at great expense and after some soul-searching, two gallons of best whisky and three pounds of chlorinated lime (which he had been using as a disinfectant in the henhouse). Presumably he expected the lime to give up its chlorine, which would then combine with carbon and hydrogen from the alcohol (C_2H_5OH). On distilling this mixture in a copper vessel, he obtained approximately one gallon of a sweet-smelling and aromatic liquid. The remainder of the spirit he prudently distilled off to use again. The affinity of the chlorine to the alcohol was so great, he noted, that it was taken up long before the distilling process was done, so it had to be watched carefully so as to know when to set aside the ethereal portion. He also found that the product could be greatly concentrated by re-distilling, when it would be caustic and 'intensely sweet and aromatic'.[7]

Guthrie, who was clearly under the impression that he had produced Dutch liquid, later wrote to Silliman:

> As the usual process of obtaining chloric ether in alcohol is both troublesome and expensive, and from its lively and invigorating effect may become an article of some value in the *Materia Medica*, I have thought a portion of your readers might be gratified with the communication of a cheap and easy process for preparing it.[8]

Silliman observed that 'Mr Guthrie's method of preparing [the alcoholic solution of chloric ether] is ingenious, economical and original . . . it is not impossible that this combination may prove curative or restorative'.[9] It is clear that Silliman also believed that Guthrie had simply devised an easier and cheaper method of making an already known compound. What Guthrie had actually made was an alcoholic solution of chloroform. While the date of this event is not recorded, it is probable that it took place quite shortly after Guthrie read Silliman's note on chloric ether.

Since Guthrie believed he was dealing with a known substance already recommended for medical use, he had no qualms about sampling it himself, and distributing bottles of it to family and friends. His object, he said, was to test the effects of the solution on healthy subjects in order to discover its probable use as a medicine. His youngest daughter, eight-year-old Cynthia, liked to run into the laboratory, dip her fingers into the tub of liquid and taste it. He seems not to have discouraged this, but on one occasion she took too much, and fell over. When he went to pick her up he found that she had fallen soundly asleep. It is probable that he simply assumed she was drunk. Later, he wrote:

> During the last six months a great number of persons have drunk the solution of chloric ether in my laboratory, not only very freely, but frequently to the point of intoxication; and so far as I have observed, it has appeared to be singularly grateful, both to the palate and stomach, producing promptly a lively flow of animal spirits, and consequent loquacity; and leaving, after its operation, little of that depression consequent to the use of ardent spirits.[10]

No wonder the locals referred to the new medicine as 'Guthrie's sweet whiskey'.[11] Indeed, that summer the citizens of Sackets Harbor were scandalised to see two of the most respectable old ladies in the town lying on the grass by the roadway apparently very drunk. Having started out to take tea with friends they had become curious about the vial of liquid one of them carried, uncorked it and inhaled it so deeply and so long that they were overcome by the vapour.

Guthrie was sure his product had great potential: 'From the invariably agreeable effects of it on persons in health, and the deliciousness of its flavour, it would seem to promise much as a remedy in cases requiring a safe, quick, energetic and palatable stimulus. For drinking, it requires an equal bulk of water.'[12]

Unfortunately the article announcing the discovery is undated, but since the preceding article is dated July 1831 and the succeeding one 2 July 1831 it is reasonable to attribute a date of 1 July to Guthrie's paper. In a later article, dated 12 September 1831, Guthrie refers to supplying Silliman with a bottle and a phial containing alcoholic solutions of chloric ether, which clearly shows that by that date Silliman knew the results of Guthrie's work.

Professor Silliman felt a few words of caution were required about the stimulating nature of the beverage, and wrote that Dr Guthrie's experiments had been '*quite sufficient*, and we ought to discountenance any other than medical use of this singular solution; unless indeed it should be found to be of utility in some of the arts. He would be no benefactor to his species, who should add a new attraction to intoxicating spirit.'[13]

Like Guthrie, Silliman was not entirely sure what had happened in the still, but he theorised that the lime had caused the alcohol to simply lose two atoms of hydrogen and one of oxygen and replace them with two of chlorine.[14] What had actually happened in the still was a lot more complicated: it was not one reaction but a series of three that had finally resulted in chloroform.[15]

In August 1831, the 22-year-old Oliver Payson Hubbard (later Professor Hubbard, and Professor Silliman's son-in-law) had entered Yale College as Silliman's assistant. Dr Guthrie had sent the college a box of his products, and among the priming powders and potato molasses were several bottles of the new distillate. It was in October 1831 that Hubbard successfully repeated Guthrie's process, a month before von Liebig completed his work.[16]

CHLORKOHLENSTOFF

Justus von Liebig was one of the great scientific pioneers of his age, revered as the father of organic chemistry. He was born in Darmstadt in 1803 where his father dealt in colours. His poor school record was the despair of his family, since his preference for experiment rather than rote learning neither endeared him to his masters nor led to academic success. At fifteen he started working for an apothecary and spent his spare time conducting experiments in his attic, and reading chemistry books. He persuaded his father to let him go to the university of Bonn where he made up for his previous neglect of his studies; in 1822, at just nineteen, he took the degree of doctor of philosophy and published his first paper. He continued his studies in Paris and made the acquaintance of many of the leading chemists of the day. In 1824 he was appointed professor at the little university of Giessen. Together with his lifelong friend and colleague, Friedrich Wöhler, he worked to develop apparatus and techniques that would vastly improve the ability of researchers to establish the chemical formulae of compounds. Publishing an average of thirty papers a year, he introduced many new compounds to chemistry.

In contrast to the calm and patient Wöhler, Liebig was rash and hot-tempered, which often led him into arguments with other chemists. He both worked and quarrelled with one of the leading chemists of the day, Professor Jean-Baptiste André Dumas. Liebig's ambition was to establish himself as a leading force in organic chemistry. He was jealous of Dumas's pre-eminence and thought that younger French chemists believed that the only important developments were happening in France. Sometimes, as even his friends and admirers admitted, his eagerness to be the first with a new discovery led him to publish his results too hastily.

In November 1831 Liebig was experimenting on the action of chlorine with alcohol, and isolated a white crystalline product. On adding an alkali he obtained a volatile liquid, which he named *chlorkohlenstoff* or 'carbon chloride'. Anxious to beat Dumas to publication, his rushed analysis had led him to miss the presence of hydrogen in the compound and he recorded that the formula was C_2Cl_5. This discovery was first referred to in a note published in the November 1831 issue of Poggendorff's *Annalen der Physik und Chemie* but the full results of his work were not published until February 1832. It still appeared, however, that Liebig, for all his eagerness, had been pre-empted by a Frenchman.

ETHER BICHLORIQUE

Eugène Soubeiran was born in Paris in 1797. To describe him simply as a pharmacist gives little impression of a most distinguished career in that field. The author of numerous treatises and manuals on pharmacy, and founder of the *Journal de Pharmacie*, he became in time the chief director of hospital pharmacies in Paris, and, in 1853, the year in which he received his doctorate, Professor of the School of Pharmacy.

On an unknown date in either late 1831 or early 1832, Soubeiran, while working on a series of experiments with chlorine compounds, distilled alcohol with bleaching powder (a mixture of chlorine compounds first made in 1799), and reported the formation of 'an ethereal liquid, very limpid and colourless, with a penetrating and very sweet odour. When breathed, the vapours which penetrate to the palate develop a taste decidedly saccharine. It may almost be said to have a saccharine odour'.[17] He called the sweet liquid *éther bichlorique* and gave it the formula CH_2Cl_2.

Soubeiran's results were published in the October 1831 issue of *Annales de Chimie et de Physique*, which appeared to give him six weeks' edge over Liebig. However, as Liebig later pointed out, because of the 1830 Revolution, the edition dated October 1831 was not published until January of the following year. It had also been clear from comments made by Soubeiran at a meeting in

November 1831 that he had not at that point discovered *éther bichlorique*. Moreover, the *Journal de Pharmacie*, of which Soubeiran was co-editor, and which one might assume would publish him as soon as possible, did not include his article until January 1832. The conclusion was that, taking into account the actual dates of publication, Liebig had got there first. Whether or not Soubeiran claimed priority during his lifetime, he continued to work on chloroform, and devised a method of preparing it that enabled it to be manufactured in large quantities. Liebig, in his efforts to prove his priority over Soubeiran, declared that his work was complete in November 1831, thus, unknown to him, settling the matter in Guthrie's favour.

CHLORIC ETHER

Meanwhile, back in Sackets Harbor, the locals had been sipping Dr Guthrie's 'sweet whiskey' for nearly a year. Silliman had repeated Guthrie's process with highly satisfactory results, but despite the fact that he, unlike Guthrie, had many years' experience of Dutch liquid, the Professor did not notice that the new product was different. This initial confusion between the two liquids meant that the solution of chloroform in alcohol eventually became popularly known as 'chloric ether'. Silliman distributed bottles of it to his medical friends, and they seemed more than happy to try it out on their patients. Dr Eli Ives, professor of medicine at Yale, wrote a number of letters to Professor Silliman in January 1832 expressing his great appreciation of 'chloric ether', which he had been using for some months. He had given it in doses of half a teaspoonful to a sixty-year-old lady with asthma, and it had produced speedy and effective relief. Another patient with lung disease had inhaled it, receiving a 'pleasant sensation'. A child with scarlet fever and an ulcerated throat received drops of the medicine diluted in water, and made a rapid recovery, while it was most beneficial in cases of spasmodic cough. Ives said he intended to use it more extensively as soon as he had a good supply.[18] His son, Dr Nathan Ives, noted its soothing effects in a case of quinsy (abscess of the throat) and pneumonia.[19]

Both doctors and patients were eager to obtain more supplies for regular use, and Silliman wrote to Guthrie asking him to prepare further supplies. Guthrie was too ill to do so from 7

October to the end of December (was he perhaps recovering from one of his explosions?), but on 24 December he replied that he was improving rapidly and hoped in a few days to be able to go into his laboratory and prepare more chloric ether, which he would forward to his agents, Van Buren, Wardell and Co. of New York. The price he named is not recorded, but Silliman approvingly thought it to be very low.

Silliman, presumably still concerned about the alcoholic effect, wondered if there was any way that the alcohol could be detached from the 'chloric ether'. Guthrie duly returned to his laboratory and was able to report on 15 February 1832 that he had succeeded in removing all the alcohol, by distillation off sulphuric acid. The slight contamination could be washed off with potassium carbonate, a strong alkali, and he now regarded the product as absolutely pure. Not only had Guthrie prepared chloroform before Liebig and Soubeiran, he had also purified it first. If at this point both Guthrie and Silliman were unaware that they had a new compound it is understandable that neither attempted to assign it a formula. It was this, rather than any medical use, that was occupying the minds of European chemists.

CHLOROFORME

Dumas believed that both Liebig and Soubeiran were incorrect in their analyses, and in 1834 he published the results of his work, which showed that *éther bichlorique* was composed of carbon, hydrogen and chlorine in the proportions of approximately 10 parts carbon to 1 of hydrogen and 89 of chlorine.[20] In 1834 there was no generally accepted table of atomic weights, and the one available to Dumas gave values to these three elements of 6, 1 and 35 respectively, which led him to the conclusion that the correct formula was C_2HCl_3. It was not until the 1860s that the atomic weight of carbon was established as 12, and many chemical formulae had to be rewritten, including that for chloroform, which only has one carbon atom.

It was this early misunderstanding, however, that gave chloroform its popular name. The prevalent theory of Dumas's day was that the building blocks of organic compounds included indivisible groupings of atoms called 'radicals'. Formic acid (HCOOH), for example, which had first been isolated in 1776 by distilling ants (family *Formicidae*), was then thought to be a combination of a formyl (sometimes spelled 'formyle' or 'formule') radical C_2H and three oxygen atoms. It appeared to Dumas that the fragrant fluid was part of this series, being composed of the formyl radical plus three chlorine atoms, and he therefore named it *chloroforme*. He made one observation about the compound that was to escape the medical profession for many years, that if the pure product was allowed to stand for a time, it became acidic, producing hydrochloric acid. Liebig, who later agreed with Dumas's analysis, called it 'perchloride of formyle'. At the time, chloroform seemed not to be of any great significance, but its later emergence as a potent anaesthetic may have prompted Liebig to make his claim for priority.

As the years passed, the commercial importance of Sackets Harbor declined, and Guthrie, who had once been regarded as a wealthy man, found that his empire was no longer of significant value. The many injuries he had suffered in explosions had damaged his health, and from his mid-fifties he was practically an invalid. He became afflicted with *tic doloureux*, a condition now known as trigeminal neuralgia, which caused stabbing pains in his face and contracted the muscles on the left side, affecting one corner of his mouth and eye. Ironically, this is one of the conditions for which chloroform was later used to afford relief. It is said that on the only occasion when a portrait was taken of him, Guthrie destroyed it with an oath, and never had another made. Certainly, no likeness of him survives. Nevertheless, his housekeeper, whom he employed in 1840 after his wife's early death, described him not unflatteringly as 'a tall fine-looking elderly gentleman with grey hair, a long beard and very piercing eyes'.[21]

Guthrie died on 19 October 1848, having seen his discovery recognised as an anaesthetic and taken up with enthusiasm by the medical profession. Local tradition has Guthrie setting fractures and performing operations on chloroformed patients, but it is stretching credulity to suggest that such a man both discovered and practised anaesthesia but neither published his work nor saw its commercial potential. It is clear from the somewhat pathetic letter he wrote to his daughter Harriet in February 1848 that he had never discovered the anaesthetic capabilities of chloroform:

> I could have made a fortune if I had gone to New York as I was urged last fall by making sweet whiskey which you remember

> taking when suffocated with charcoal. You see it called Chloroform and the newspapers are beginning to give the credit of discovering it. I made the first particle that was ever made and you are the first human being that ever used it in sickness. This is likely to prove the grandest discovery in medicine the world ever saw. By breathing it a few seconds the person falls apparently into a sweet sleep – when breasts legs and arms may be cut away – painful labours ended and all without pain or injury.[22]

In 1888 a committee of the Chicago Medical Society was appointed to examine the rival claims and concluded that the discoverer of chloroform was Dr Samuel Guthrie. Credit to Guthrie was also given in the *Apotheker Zeitung* of Berlin in 1893, while in 1894 the *London Chemist* additionally credited Guthrie with being the first to produce pure chloroform.

For nearly sixteen years after its discovery, chloroform languished as a chemical curiosity in the laboratories of Europe. It was not in the pharmacopoeias and very few journals even mentioned its existence. Due to Dr Guthrie's work and the support of Professor Silliman, it was better known in the United States, where 'chloric ether', a 12 per cent solution of chloroform in alcohol, was occasionally used as a carminative. It was eventually awarded a mention in the *United States Dispensatory*, which praised its 'bland sweet taste' and ease of administration to children:

> It has been used with advantage in asthma, spasmodic cough, the sore throat of scarlet fever, atonic quinsy, and other diseases in which a grateful and composing medicine is indicated. In affections characterised by difficult respiration, it may be used by inhalation.[23]

The introduction of chloroform as an anaesthetic was to happen not in the USA but the United Kingdom, and was the culmination of a series of unconnected events that took place in Liverpool, London and Edinburgh. In the late 1830s, a prescription was brought into the Apothecaries Hall in Liverpool (possibly by an American visitor), an ingredient of which was chloric ether, but no one there knew what it was. Dr Brett, the company chemist, did some investigation and found the reference in the United States Dispensatory, which included a formula for its preparation. He made some, and it was later prescribed by Liverpool doctors, notably Richard Formby.

Morton's triumphant introduction of ether anaesthesia in 1846 prompted the investigation of similar substances as potential anaesthetics. Chloric ether was tried by Bigelow but abandoned as not sufficiently effective. In London, Mr Tomes, a dentist at the Middlesex Hospital, also tried and abandoned it after extracting a molar from a patient who was furious with him afterwards, as she had been conscious but unable to move throughout the operation.[24] Jacob Bell, pharmacist at the Middlesex, reported in February 1847, 'Chloric ether has been tried in some cases with success, it is more pleasant to the taste, but appears to be rather less powerful in its effects than sulphuric ether.'[25]

In May 1847, a seventeen-year-old medical student at the Middlesex, Michael Cudmore (later Professor) Furnell, fascinated by ether and its selection of inhalers, started amusing himself with some personal experiments.[26] Bell, who was his tutor, anxiously forbade him access to ether. Undeterred, Furnell searched the storeroom for some other likely intoxicating substance, discovered a neglected bottle labelled 'chloric ether', found that it smelled pleasant, put some in an instrument, and proceeded to inhale it. Not only did it begin to induce insensibility, but it did so without the bronchial irritation which he knew made ether impossible for some patients to tolerate. Furnell at once mentioned this to Bell, who recommended that he take it to St Bartholomew's Hospital. There, Furnell showed it to Dr Holmes Coote, who cautiously asked him if he could guarantee its safety. Furnell replied confidently that he knew it was safe, because he had tried it on himself and was none the worse. This was obviously good enough for Coote, who, with a Dr Lawrence, used it on a patient the very same day. Like Bell, they found that the results were unpredictable, so they tried using it combined with the same volume of ether,[27] and this continued throughout the summer and autumn of 1847.

It was a worthy effort, but the medical profession was understandably unimpressed, and most were unaware that 'chloric ether' was simply diluted chloroform. If they had known, they might have heeded the advice of French physiologist Marie Jean Pierre Flourens, who, in February and March 1847 conducted experiments on animals using pure chloroform, and discovered that inhalation led to insensibility. Recognising the potential power of chloroform, he recommended that it was too dangerous to use on humans.[28]

By then, Dr Brett had been succeeded at Apothecaries Hall by David Waldie. A native of Linlithgow, he qualified as a doctor in Edinburgh, where he had made the acquaintance of James Simpson, and later turned to pharmacy as a profession. Waldie found that Brett's method of manufacturing chloric ether resulted in a product of variable strength with some unpleasant impurities. Accordingly he introduced a new process, separating and purifying the chloroform, then dissolving it in pure spirit. His interest in and knowledge of the chemistry of chloric ether was to have dramatic consequences.

THREE

ADAM'S RIB

> I have no doubt of some physiological and therefore needful and useful connection of the pain and the powers of parturition, the inconveniences of which are really less considerable than has by some been supposed.
>
> *Charles D. Meigs, Professor of Midwifery and Diseases of Women and Children, Jefferson Medical College, Philadelphia, 1848*[1]

In October 1869, before a large assembly of distinguished ladies and gentlemen, Sir James Young Simpson, Baronet, professor of midwifery, was awarded the freedom of the City of Edinburgh. It was, said the Lord Provost, a 'token of very great respect and admiration'. Simpson's reputation was 'known over the whole civilized world' for he had made 'the greatest of all discoveries in modern times in connection with medicine'.[2] The Lord Provost was referring to events twenty-two years previously, when Simpson had secured his status as a national hero with a series of crude and hazardous experiments that revealed the extraordinary power of chloroform.

His beginnings were humble and this, at a time when class barriers were more rarely crossed than now, made his achievements all the more remarkable. He was born on 7 June 1811, in Bathgate, near Edinburgh, the seventh son and eighth child of a baker. On the day of his birth, the doctor's fee was greater than the takings in his father's shop.

A small, sturdy boy with an over-large head, James showed his intellectual promise from an early age, and at a time when many families could only afford to send one child to higher education, if that, the 'wise wean', as he was known, was the obvious candidate. Simpson started school at four, and went to Edinburgh University at the age of fourteen. Originally destined for an arts course, he lodged with medical students whose books and conversation aroused his interest, and he soon transferred to the study of medicine. He was in exactly the right place. Edinburgh was one of the leading medical schools in the world, and the first in the United Kingdom to have a chair of midwifery. Against considerable opposition, its professor, James Hamilton, had established midwifery, once regarded as a study unworthy of a gentleman, as a required subject for medical qualification. However, Simpson did not initially find midwifery the most interesting of subjects: tired from his long hours of study, he regularly dozed during Professor Hamilton's lectures. It may have been during this part of his life that he was so frequently referred to as 'Young Simpson' that he later adopted 'Young' as his middle name.

He was a striking young man, his large head framed by a mass of long tangled auburn hair. The flat, coarse-featured face can never have been attractive, but there were lively eyes under the heavy brows, and a surprisingly delicate mouth. The stocky body was destined to become decidedly rounded in later life, and his hands were broad and powerful, though the fingers tapered and were unexpectedly sensitive of touch.

His first, distressing sight of surgery had made him acutely conscious of the horrors of pain, and he later wrote of 'that great principle of emotion which both impels us to feel sympathy at the sight of suffering in any fellow creature, and at the same time imparts to us delight and gratification in the exercise of any power by which we can mitigate and alleviate that suffering.'[3] Simpson, who freely admitted that he was never able to get into the dentist's chair without 'the stimulus to my courage . . . of two or three glasses of whisky',[4] declared, 'All pain is *per se* and especially in excess, destructive and even ultimately fatal in its action and effects.'[5]

Simpson received his MD in 1831. He was clearly not destined to be a surgeon, but it was not until 1833 that he became interested in midwifery, and made up for his earlier neglect by attending regular lectures. In 1835 he was elected one of the annual presidents of the Royal Medical Society. His inaugural address was well received, as were his publications, and his reputation and clinical practice grew rapidly. His patients found him both charming and sympathetic. The *Lancet* said of him: 'His winning manners, his power of entering fully and at once into the mind and heart of the patient . . . wonderfully reinforced his professional sagacity and skill.'[6] His house soon became crowded with patients whom he treated according to their need rather than their ability to pay. After the financial struggles of his youth, finding that he now had sufficient to live on, he cared little about money. The relief of pain was never far from his mind. 'Cannot something be done to render the patient unconscious while under acute pain, without interfering with the free and healthy play of natural functions?' he wrote to a fellow doctor in 1836,[7] and in the following year he experimented with mesmerism. By then midwifery was his preferred field and he spent a year working at a lying-in hospital to gain further experience, becoming a lecturer in midwifery in 1838.

There was another, less affable side to Simpson, which his friends readily acknowledged. He had strong feelings, and spoke plainly, sometimes harshly. In 1839 his promising career nearly came to an abrupt halt, when he commented to a Dr Lewins, 'That was a scandalous and lying article in the *Observer*. I hope you were not the author of it?'[8] As it so happened, Lewins was, and matters reached the point where the preliminaries of a duel were being arranged, but three mutual friends intervened and smoothed things over. This was only one of numerous professional squabbles that littered his career.

When Professor Hamilton resigned the chair of midwifery in 1839, Simpson applied. He had two serious rivals for the place, and also two drawbacks, his youth – he was only twenty-eight – and the fact that he was a bachelor. The first he could do nothing about, but fortunately he had a long-established understanding with a cousin, Jessie Grindlay, and they were soon married. Simpson went into debt to spend the then huge sum of £500 on his campaign, and when the election took place he won by one vote. Immediately afterwards the happy couple departed on honeymoon.

The new professor's classes soon became extremely popular: 'the forcible and lucid style . . . his breadth of view . . . the pleasant talk and sallies of quiet humour with which he often relieved the dry exposition . . . all conduced to make him a favourite of the students generally'.[9] Soon, it was standing room only for his lectures, and demand became so great that eventually he had to apply for extra sessions.[10] The professorship also resulted in a rapid expansion of his clinical practice, and a new social class of patient. 'I have made a bargain for a carriage. . . . I saw yesterday one Viscountess and three "Ladies"', he wrote to his brother in 1840. 'Good for one day among the nobility.'[11]

He did not, however, forget his humble origins. Walter Channing, a visiting obstetrician from the United States, later wrote about his stay and described how the house was always crowded with patients of all classes, who drew lots for the order in which they saw Simpson: 'Here are the poor and rich together. There is no difference in their treatment.'[12]

By 1845, the floods of patients and a growing family necessitated a move to 52 Queen Street, Edinburgh, where he was to live for the rest of his life. The house always seemed to be bustling, as visitors were constantly arriving and often ended up staying to dinner. His hospitality became well known: 'at each meal his table was surrounded by a strange medley of guests, distinguished foreigners, tourists, and patients',[13] and the chaotic household arrangements were supervised by the ever patient and supportive Jessie.

Simpson was a man of enormous and unfailing energy, and tremendous breadth of interests, once described by Dr John Brown of Edinburgh as 'overwhelmed with work as ever, and plunging about rejoicing in it, like any seal in the Bay of Baffin.'[14] He regularly travelled considerable distances for meetings and consultations. In 1847 Simpson described a trip to London where he 'breakfasted with the Secretary of War, dined with the Mistress of the Robes, and had tea and an egg with the Premier'. He then went to an evening discussion society where he found 'all the crack doctors . . . busy speaking against me and my published opinions. I was driven to speak in self-defence and set them right.'[15]

Simpson needed very little driving to set people right, and indeed this comment may well have been self-mocking. His friend and biographer John Duns wrote of him, 'when Dr Simpson took up a well-defined position in a controversy, he held it bravely against all comers. When convinced that he was right, he was utterly immovable. Neither argument nor appeal could lead him to change his views.'[16] Simpson would often go into print to ridicule those who disagreed with him, which he attributed to prejudice, blindness or simple stupidity. 'In the advocacy or defence of new methods of treatment, or of new remedies, he seldom took into account the prejudices or even the honest convictions of others', wrote Duns, adding 'he often trampled on the long-cherished convictions of professional brethren, and in consequence made many enemies.'[17]

When Simpson heard of ether being used in London he at once went there to see it for himself, and spent Christmas 1846 as the guest of his old tutor Robert Liston, who had been professor of clinical surgery at University College London since 1835. On 21 December an enthralled audience at University College Hospital saw a butler named Frederic Churchill given ether before Liston amputated his leg. The patient felt nothing, and Liston commented, 'This Yankee dodge, gentlemen, beats mesmerism hollow!'[18] The operation had taken 28 seconds.

Ether was soon the new medical wonder. On 4 January 1847 readers of *The Times* were regaled with a detailed description of the amputation of a leg in Bristol; the etherised patient awoke 'perfectly quiet and calm, and said he had not felt any pain'.[19] By 13 January the journal of the Pharmaceutical Society, whose members had already devised ten different ether inhalers, stated, 'This is now the all-engrossing subject, and the public attention is daily called to the several operations which have been performed without the accompaniment of the severe pain heretofore experienced.'[20] It seemed that surgery under ether could even be enjoyable. An Irishman having his leg removed entertained the onlookers with humorous observations, nods and winks, and declared afterwards that he had had 'most pleasurable sensations', while a woman felt transported to 'a beautiful heaven' and cried with delight to find her operation painlessly over.[21] For a patient dreading surgery, it must have seemed like a dream come true.

It was Liston's opinion that ether would only be safe for short operations. Simpson, however, naturally hopeful of its potential in obstetrics, returned to Edinburgh keen to demonstrate that ether could be used for longer procedures. He first used ether on 19 January 1847, in a midwifery case where the patient had a deformed pelvis. There was no hope for the child and grave risk to the mother. To Simpson's delight, the mother suffered no pain and survived the complicated delivery. Coincidentally, on the same day he received a letter appointing him Queen's Physician in Scotland; but when he wrote to his brother, it was the painless delivery that most excited him, and he confessed, 'I can think of naught else.'[22] Simpson continued to use ether, not only for complicated labour but also, more controversially, for natural labour, collecting statistics to prove that it increased survival rates. He soon concluded, however, that ether's smell and irritant properties made it less than ideal, and began to look for something better.

In the meantime, Simpson had to consider the views of his opponents. One objector to anaesthesia, Dr James Pickford, declared, on no grounds other than his preconceived notions, that 'pain in surgical operations is in a majority of cases even desirable, and its prevention or annihilation is for the most part hazardous to the patient'.[23] Simpson also received letters from obstetricians who, while happy about the relief of surgical pain, believed that the pain of childbirth was part of a natural function which must have a useful purpose. These early clashes meant that when, a year later, Simpson needed to fly to the defence of his own discovery, his arguments were already well thought-out.

Since Morton's demonstration, the safety of ether had not been seriously called into question, but it soon appeared that Faraday's words of caution in 1818 were not misplaced. Less than three months after the introduction of ether in the United Kingdom, the high hopes of both surgeons and patients were to be shattered. Ann Parkinson of Grantham, who was just twenty-one, had a large, possibly malignant growth on her thigh, but had understandably hesitated about suffering the ordeal of surgery. Early in 1847 she read about ether in the newspapers and asked her doctor if he would use it for an operation. Surgery took place on 9 March, and was successful, but she was left in a weakened state from which she never rallied, and died two days later. The inquest attached no blame to the doctor, and death was put down to the inhalation of ether. This event must have increased Simpson's resolve to find another agent, with all the advantages of ether but none of its faults.

Simpson was by then a widely published authority on obstetrics; when Queen Victoria, in the January of that year, conferred upon him the post of Physician Accoucheur to the Queen for Scotland, she had referred to 'his high character and abilities'.[24] But the man of high character was about to embark on a very dubious enterprise.

By modern standards, Simpson's experiments in search of a better anaesthetic seem both unscientific and alarmingly dangerous. His method was simply to acquire samples of any substances that might have a breatheable vapour, inhale them from a tumbler, and make notes of his reactions. The experiments continued throughout the summer and autumn of 1847, and he later reported that, before lighting on chloroform, he had found three other substances which would also cause anaesthesia, but with such unpleasant side-effects that he could not recommend their use.[25]

Ethyl nitrate, nowadays an ingredient of perfumes, dyes and rocket propellant, was easy and pleasant to inhale, and a rapid and powerful anaesthetic, but led to noises and a sense of fullness in the head, followed by headaches and giddiness. Benzin (*sic*), nowadays used as an industrial solvent, is highly toxic and a known carcinogen. The ringing noises in the head after inhalation were almost intolerable. Carbon disulphide is an explosive chemical once widely used as a soil fumigant. This was an effective anaesthetic, but resulted in visions, headaches and giddiness. It also smelled like rotten cabbage. Simpson tried and rejected acetone, which is domestically familiar to us as nail polish remover, and will certainly cause unconsciousness if inhaled, but will also damage the lungs, and iodoform, another toxic chemical. Dutch liquid caused such great irritation of the throat, that few people could go on breathing it for long.

These inhalations were carried out around the dining-table of 52 Queen Street, either in the morning or the late evening, when Simpson was usually accompanied by his assistants, Dr George Keith and Dr J. Matthews Duncan. Professor James Miller, a surgeon who was a friend and close neighbour, took an interest and would call in from time to time, to see what progress had been made, and possibly also to check if Simpson was all right. These experiments must have caused some disquiet in the Simpson household, as well as a resigned acceptance of the complete uselessness of trying to dissuade him.

In October 1847 Simpson's old friend David Waldie paid him a visit, and Simpson took the opportunity to pick his brains about likely anaesthetics. Waldie, being both a doctor and a chemist, was in a unique position to offer advice. During the course of the conservation, Simpson mentioned chloric ether. He had been introduced to it by his friend, Dr Richard Formby, and he may also, through travel and correspondence, have known of the experiments at St Bartholomew's and the Middlesex Hospital, but he was not, as Waldie discovered, aware that it was simply a solution of chloroform. He advised Simpson to try pure chloroform, and offered to supply some on his return to Liverpool. Unfortunately, due to a fire at his laboratory (either during the visit or shortly afterwards – the precise date is unknown) he was unable to fulfil his promise. But Simpson managed to obtain a chloroform sample locally. It didn't look promising. The heaviness of the liquid, nearly one and a half times the specific gravity of water, was not suggestive of something that would vaporise easily, and he set it aside.

On the evening of 4 November 1847 Drs Simpson, Keith and Duncan sat down in the dining-room for their regular experiments. Other members of the family were also present, including Mrs Simpson, her sister Miss Grindlay, her niece Miss Petrie and Captain Petrie, a brother-in-law. A number of substances having been tried without effect, Simpson recalled the bottle of chloroform on a side table, and after some searching, found it under a heap of paper. A small amount was poured into each tumbler and the doctors began to inhale. Almost at once a curious hilarity came over them, and they exclaimed on the delicious aroma of the fluid. The bright-eyed young doctors became extremely talkative, and it seemed to them that their conversation was unusually intelligent and charming to their listeners. In other words, they were drunk.

Simpson's next thought was, 'This is far stronger and better than ether.' His second thought was to notice that he was lying on the floor staring up at the ceiling, and there was much confusion and alarm all around him. As he later described it, 'We all inhaled the fluid and we were all under the mahogany in a trice.'[26]

Looking around for his colleagues, he saw Dr Duncan lying under a chair, jaw sagging, eyes staring, head dropped to his chest, unconscious and snoring in an alarmingly determined manner. Hearing a thumping noise, Simpson turned to Dr Keith, and saw him lying under the table, his legs thrashing as if he was trying to overturn it. As Keith gradually ceased to kick he raised his head to the level of the table and stared with unconscious eyes, the ghastliness of his expression creating a terror in Miss Grindlay that she was to speak of for many years to come. With some effort, Simpson was able to get back into his chair and Duncan and Keith slowly awoke and were again seated. All three were so delighted that they at once decided to try it again. They inhaled chloroform several more times, though not to the point of unconsciousness. Miss Petrie was determined to try it, too, and sitting at the table, she inhaled deeply, folded her arms across her breast and fell asleep crying, 'I'm an angel! Oh I'm an angel!'[27]

Once the supply was used up, the doctors continued eagerly discussing the experiment. All were agreed that they had found something far better than ether, not only more effective, but much pleasanter to inhale. It was 3 a.m. before the happy party broke up, but the following morning they lost no time in contacting a manufacturing chemist.

The fortunate firm was Duncan and Flockhart. The hard-working partners agreed to supply Simpson with the chloroform, and laboured into the small hours of the morning to supply what was demanded. Four pounds of chloride of lime, 12 lb of water, and 12 ounces of spirit were placed in a large still and heated gently. After a violent frothing reaction the material separated into two layers, the lower being chloroform and the upper, weak spirit. These were separated out and the alkaline residues removed with sulphuric acid. Barium carbonate was added to remove any traces of acid, then it was left to stand with quicklime, as the reaction with the residual water would dry the product. It was now possible to re-distil what promised to be almost pure chloroform. Simpson must have awaited the result with some impatience. It would have been two or even three days before he was able to collect his order, and he lost no time in using it.

His first recorded medical use of chloroform was on 8 November 1847, in an obstetric case. Jane Carstairs was in her second pregnancy, the first having ended with a three-day labour and the death of the child. She was therefore very anxious, and had slept little in the previous two nights. Simpson rolled a handkerchief into a cone, moistened it with half a teaspoonful of chloroform, and placed it over her mouth and nostrils. Twenty-five minutes later, the child was born safely. The nurse took the child into the next room, and some while later the new mother awoke, saying she had enjoyed a refreshing sleep, which she had needed to be more able for the work ahead. Simpson deliberately did not comment, and a few moments later she said she was afraid that the chloroform had stopped the pains. When Simpson asked the nurse to bring the infant to her, the new mother took some convincing that labour was indeed over, and this was 'her own living baby'.[28]

The first patient to receive chloroform for tooth extraction was T.D. Morrison, the apprentice of Edinburgh dentist Francis Imlach, who after agreeing to the test wrote a letter to Simpson freeing him from any responsibility in the case of accident. A number of scientific observers were present at Simpson's house for the procedure, which took place on 10 November, and was a great success.[29] Fired with enthusiasm, Simpson was now eager to use chloroform in surgical cases, and Professor Miller agreed that chloroform could be administered to his patients in the Edinburgh Royal Infirmary. The first scheduled operation was for a strangulated hernia, but in the event Simpson could not be present and chloroform was not used. The operation proceeded without an anaesthetic and the patient died suddenly on the table after the first incision. Simpson was later to observe that, had this been his first case, chloroform would have been blamed for the death, impeding the progress of anaesthesia. He was able to attend on 12 November when Miller had three patients awaiting surgery. The first was a little boy or four or five who spoke only Gaelic, and was operated on to remove the diseased radius bone of his forearm. After being held and made to inhale chloroform from a handkerchief, he fell into a snoring sleep and the operation was performed successfully.

'Half an hour afterwards,' stated Miller, 'he was found in bed, like a child newly awakened from a refreshing sleep, with a clear merry eye, and placid expression of countenance, wholly unlike what is found to obtain after ordinary etherisation.'[30]

The second operation was on the face of a soldier, who was given chloroform on a sponge, and so approved of it that when he came to he thrust the sponge into his mouth and happily continued inhaling. The third patient was a young man requiring amputation of a toe. Many medical men were present to witness these operations, among them the French chemist Dumas, who happened to be passing through Edinburgh at the time. The following day a young woman came to Miller's house for removal of a tumour from her jaw. She inhaled the chloroform from a sponge, and fell asleep seated in a chair. Miller was impressed with 'her manageableness during the operation . . . as perfect as if she had been a wax doll'.[31]

The next few days were a flurry of activity. Simpson used chloroform on up to thirty individuals, and wrote a paper for publication in the *Lancet*. With an affection for the material that caused him to seriously misrepresent its qualities, he described chloroform as possessing 'an agreeable, fragrant, fruit-like odour, and a saccharine, pleasant taste'[32] thus making it sound no more dangerous than a glass of orange juice. He was more accurate in listing its advantages. Only 100 to 120 drops, and sometimes far less, were sufficient to produce the anaesthetic effect; the action was rapid, complete and more persistent than ether. Not only did this save time for the surgeon, but the period of initial excitement was practically abolished. It was less expensive and more portable than ether, and altogether pleasanter and easier to use. Well aware that obstetricians would oppose the use of anaesthesia, he made a point of declaring that since using it he had never seen better or more rapid recoveries, and never witnessed any unpleasant results to either mother or child.

Once Simpson had set out his stall, he was never to retreat. The advantages of chloroform were to him so self-evident that anyone who opposed its use was either hidebound by old dogmas or a fool. Nothing was to be permitted to stand in the way of the universal acceptance of this great boon to mankind. Simpson brought to the fight his considerable authority and his popularity with patients, and brushed aside caution, doubt and outright opposition with vigour, humour and relish. The force of his confident personality, and his active publicising of the discovery were powerful factors in the rapid spread of the news and the conversion of the medical profession to chloroform.

Simpson sent his article to the *Lancet* in time for the 21 November edition, but he wanted a wider audience than the medical profession. He also wrote a pamphlet, 'On a New Anaesthetic Agent, More Efficient Than Sulphuric Ether', that included Miller's rapturous descriptions of the operations. Simpson did not forget the contribution of his friend, David Waldie, and sent him a reprint of the paper with the comment, 'I am sure you will be delighted to see part of the good results of our hasty conversation.'[33] The pamphlet was published on 17 November, price 6*d*, and advertised on the front page of that day's *Scotsman*.

By 27 November it was reported that 1,500 copies had been sold.[34] There was an immediate demand for chloroform, and chemists all over England and Scotland were obliged to labour through the night to fulfil the flood of orders. Simpson sent copies of the pamphlet to leading members of the medical profession all over the world, and his easily accessible style meant that it was also widely read by the public. There was a not unnatural fear that patients would take matters into their own hands and demand chloroform anaesthesia from their doctors, and in many cases this was exactly what happened. Professor Montgomery of the Dublin medical school wrote to Simpson saying that copies of Simpson's pamphlet had been 'most industriously circulated though every class in this city . . . in which pamphlets many things are submitted to the perusal of the public which in my judgement were better withheld.'[35]

Those doctors who had used ether were keen to try chloroform at once. On 17 November, Liston wrote to Professor Miller, 'The "chloroform" is a vast advance upon ether. I have tried it with perfect success . . . Simpson deserves all laudation.'[36] There was some concern about the tendency of patients to vomit, but Francis Imlach, driving the first wedge into the English/Scottish divide, was scathing of London methods and declared that vomiting was entirely due to using impure chloroform or applying it incorrectly.[37]

On 15 December, members of the committee formed in Edinburgh at Simpson's instigation only three weeks previously made a report after a series of experiments on animals, students, and of course, themselves. The unanimous conclusion was that ether should be abandoned in favour of chloroform. 'On some points,' it was recorded, 'the report of the committee had been superseded by the decision of the profession at large. There was no instance on record where the discovery of a remedy had been so rapidly made known and its employment so universally adopted as that of the inhalation of chloroform.'[38]

There was a charm in the breezy simplicity of Simpson's instructions. Doctors were freed from awkward and expensive inhalers – Simpson dismissed them as not only unnecessary but frightening to patients, and his applicator of choice was the plain silk handkerchief. At first he advised measuring the quantity used, suggesting an initial application of between one and three fluid drachms (a drachm being one-eighth of an ounce, or about 4 ml), but before long was declaring that he no longer did so, judging by the effect and not the amount. If the patient was not affected in a minute or so, he simply added a little more. The best test of insensibility, he advised, was a noisy, stertorous respiration. Much later it was recognised that stertorous breathing was a sign of the deepest state of insensibility, beyond which there was a danger of asphyxia, and doctors learned to avoid it. Simpson himself soon realised that a lighter anaesthesia was sufficient for obstetric cases and often applied as little as half a drachm. After the initial application, he was happy to entrust the handkerchief to the nurse or the patient's husband, teaching them to apply it when the pains returned. Sometimes, with the patient lying quietly on her side, it would be placed on the pillow by her cheek.

While the journals and newspapers were full of reports of successful operations under chloroform and its advantages over ether, there was some jealousy. Dr Bigelow of Boston, in particular, was most unhappy about the belief which had become common that Simpson had invented anaesthesia. There were those who tried to steal some of the glory for themselves. One such was a promising young doctor, Robert Mortimer Glover of Newcastle, who had published a prize-winning essay in 1842.[39] Glover had injected a number of compounds including chloroform into the veins and body cavities of dogs and rabbits, most of which had died in slow agony, and he observed that the chloroformed animals did not move when he pinched or pricked their limbs. On 14 November he wrote angrily to Simpson accusing him of ignoring his paper. Simpson knew nothing and cared less about Glover's paper, and dismissed his claim with searing contempt.[40] In Paris, some journals claimed priority for the French physiologist Flourens, on the basis of his animal experiments. On 29 November 1847, David Waldie read a modest paper to the Liverpool Literary and Philosophical Society, describing his October conversation with Simpson. He waited to receive the due recognition for his contribution to medical history, but he waited in vain. Whenever Simpson did mention him, he made light of the matter, suggesting that Waldie had simply mentioned chloroform as a possibility, rather than making a positive and knowledgeable recommendation. Waldie was not a man to make a fuss, and in 1852 he departed for a post as a commercial chemist in Calcutta. It was left to his brother to publicise his claims in 1870.[41]

While most doctors welcomed the use of chloroform in surgery, many believed that it had no place in natural labour. Dr Parke of Liverpool was astonished and appalled to find that Simpson recommended using it in all midwifery cases. Shortly after Simpson made his dramatic announcement about chloroform, he discovered that Parke was due to read a paper at the meeting of the Liverpool Medical Institution called 'On the Moral propriety of Medical men recommending the inhalation of Aether in other than extraordinary cases'. On 14 November Simpson wrote to Waldie:

> Imlach tells me Dr P. is to enlighten your medical society about the 'morality' of the practice. I have a great itching to run up and pound him. *When* is the meeting? The true moral question is, 'is a practitioner justified by *any* principles of humanity in not using it?' I believe every operation without it is just a piece of the most deliberate and cold-blooded *cruelty*. He will be at the primary curse, no doubt. But the word translated 'sorrow' is truly 'labour', 'toil'; and in the very next verse the very same word means this.[42]

There had been a few objections to ether based on the Biblical curse on Eve, but they cannot have been either numerous or serious since Simpson had not published any rebuttal. Early in 1847, Professor Miller had discussed the matter with the Reverend Dr Chalmers, Moderator of the Free Church of Scotland, who had advised that any who took this view were 'small theologians' and advised Miller to take no heed of them.

This time it was different; this time Simpson was defending his cherished chloroform, and he decided to get his retaliation in first. Before he had even seen Parke's paper, which in the event was on medical ethics, and did not mention the primary curse, Simpson had gone into print with a pamphlet entitled *Answer to the Religious Objections Advanced Against the Employment of Anaesthetic Agents in Midwifery and Surgery*.

The existence of this pamphlet has always suggested that the use of anaesthesia brought about a storm of religious opposition that Simpson triumphantly defeated, and Scottish Calvinists have been accused of denouncing chloroform from the pulpit, yet there is no evidence of any such thing. A detailed examination of the periodicals of the time made by A.D. Farr revealed only seven references to the issue, none of them in opposition.[43] Simpson did receive private communications from clergy, doctors and patients. One letter from a clergyman denounced chloroform as 'a decoy of Satan, apparently offering to bless woman; but, in the end it will harden society and rob God of the deep earnest cries, which arise in time of trouble for help'.[44]

In *Answer to the Religious Objections* Simpson clearly enjoys using rhetoric, sarcasm, humour, and the results of mugging up on Biblical Hebrew to trounce every objection that could possibly be raised. There was nothing he enjoyed more than setting up an opponent for the precise purpose of knocking him down again. He believed that the Dublin medical school had publicly denounced his conduct, as an attempt to contravene the decrees of providence which was 'hence heretical and reprehensible, and to be avoided by all properly principled students and practitioners', on the grounds that 'the Almighty had seen fit to allot pain to natural labour'.[45] Presumably, responded Simpson, no one in Dublin used carriages to avert the fatigue which the Almighty had allotted to natural walking. These comments caused considerable annoyance to Professor Montgomery, who wrote to Simpson protesting that he had never made any of the statements attributed to him.[46]

Simpson also touched a few nerves by arguing that the Lord Himself had practised anaesthesia when removing Adam's rib. 'Putting aside the impiety of making Jehovah an operating surgeon, and the absurdity of supposing that anaesthesia would be necessary in His hands,' retorted a Dr Ashwell, 'Dr Simpson surely forgets that the deep sleep of Adam took place before the introduction of pain into the world, during his state of innocence.'[47] Not many thought like Ashwell, and six months after publishing his pamphlet Simpson was able to congratulate himself on the cessation of all religious objections.

Just as the news about ether had crossed the Atlantic to England by fast steamer less than a year previously, so English and Scottish doctors sent letters to their American colleagues about the use of chloroform. Dr W.J. Little, a surgeon of the London Hospital, wrote to Dr Buckminster Brown of Boston:

> The facility and rapidity with which the effect is produced, the absence of annoyance to the inhalers and bystanders, the tranquil manner in which a person who has inhaled recovers from the state of insensibility and the length of time he remains insensible, even after inhaling the chloroform only thirty or thirty-five seconds gives it prominent advantage over ether.[48]

William Morton was still in the throes of trying to make his fortune out of ether when he received a letter from Simpson, who provided him not only with details of his work on chloroform but the formula for its preparation. Morton determined to try it at once. He and his assistant were just about to start heating the mixture when a patient 'opportunely arrived' for the purpose of having three teeth extracted under ether. 'With a little trouble,' wrote Morton, 'she was persuaded to remain until there was sufficient quantity of chloroform distilled for the experiment.'[49] Morton used a whole ounce of chloroform on his ether sponge, and the teeth were extracted without pain, and, miraculously, without killing the patient.

Before the end of 1847, established manufacturers were unable to keep up with demand, and new firms were springing up to cash in on the rush. Those with less experience of the process were unprepared for the power of the initial frothing reaction, which threatened to blow the head off the still if insufficient headspace was given, and there were a few narrow escapes.[50]

By January 1848 Simpson was writing to Professor Meigs, an influential obstetrician of Philadelphia, declaring that most or all of his brethren used chloroform, and the ladies themselves insisted on it. It had also been 'a common amusement in drawing-room parties for the last two or three months'.[51] The *risqué* details of these evenings sometimes found their way into the press:

> A practice has assumed the form of a mania in Edinburgh. . . . A number of ladies and gentlemen were invited to an evening party in the house of a respectable medical practitioner. At ten, instead of music and dancing, the learned doctor entered with flask and sponge, and every guest was treated to a trip to the realms of insensibility. Some of the ladies were foolish enough, while there, to utter such speeches as 'Oh! My beloved Charles, come to my arms!' at the same time unwittingly extending them to receive the dear creature.[52]

This learned doctor may have been none other than Simpson himself. Lady Priestley, the widow of an Edinburgh physician, later recalled Simpson's after-dinner entertainments at her parents' house when she was a girl:

> . . . the professor used to try his experiments with chloroform on us girls. He was then just introducing it, and with some of the liquid simply poured on a handkerchief, would have half a dozen of us lying about in various stages of sleep. Our mother feared nothing, and was only too delighted to sacrifice, if unavoidable, a daughter or two to science![53]

Simpson's relaxed attitude to his fruit-flavoured miracle was legendary. His sister-in-law, Miss Grindlay, had never quite got over the horrors of 4 November, and afterwards Simpson used to tease her that he would chloroform her, and chase her around the house with a bottle. He was soon overtaken with fits of laughter and she always got away. On one occasion Simpson had an effervescing drink made up of chloric ether and aerated water and served it to his dinner party guests as 'chloroform champagne'. The ladies and gentlemen tasted the drink and found it pleasant but 'heady'. Clarke, the butler, was asked to take it back down to the kitchen, where he suggested the cook try some. She was less cautious, and after drinking a glassful, collapsed. Clarke panicked and rushed upstairs yelling, 'For God's sake, sir, come down, I've poisoned the cook!' Everyone raced downstairs to find the cook lying on the kitchen floor snoring loudly, Clarke explaining he had given her a drink of the 'champagne chlory'. Everyone except Clarke and the cook laughed heartily.[54]

Dr Ashwell, who opposed obstetric anaesthesia on the grounds that chloroform deprived women of moral control, wrote to the *Lancet* to complain about 'professors . . . of our ancient universities going about from one city to another to announce and exhibit the wonderful effects of a new gas, and . . . somewhat after the manner of a showman, to demonstrate them personally at dinner parties and in drawing rooms'.[55] Simpson replied personally: '. . . my blood feels chilled by the cruel inhumanity and deliberate cruelty which you and some members of the profession openly avow . . . you have not yet had time to get rid of some old professional caprices and nonsensical thought.' He then went on to invite Ashwell to come and stay with him, promising a hearty Scotch welcome; 'and I will readily convince you how utterly you are in error on all points'.[56] Knowing what drinks were served with dinner, it seems unlikely that he accepted.

Simpson wrote this letter from his sickbed, for despite the success of chloroform, he was continuing his experiments, using himself as a subject. 'I have been laid up for the last twenty hours in bed,' he wrote, 'ill and quite undone for the time, from breathing and inhaling some vapours I was experimenting upon last night, with a view of obtaining other therapeutic agents to be used by inhalation . . .'.

Clarke, who was a great believer in 'chlory', once found his master unconscious on the floor after an experiment, and feared that he would kill himself one day. Shaking his head, he would declare his master to be a fool, for 'they'll never find anything better than chlory'.[57]

CHLOROFORM CONQUERS THE WORLD

The news of chloroform spread rapidly, in letters, journals and newspapers. In France it quickly replaced ether, and after a brief flirtation with inhalers, the general mode of administration became the simple folded cloth. There were a few detractors. In January 1848, a M. Malgaigne reported on the chloroform question to the *Academie de Medecine* in Paris. He had for some years been on terms of animosity with M. Jules Guérin, editor of the *Gazette Médicale*, who took the opportunity to attack every conclusion in his report. Ultimately, one of the parties (it is not reported which) challenged the other to a duel, but the other was wise enough to refuse it, so avoiding what might have been the first chloroform fatality.[58]

In Germany, surgeon Johann Heyfelder of Erlangen, who used chloroform successfully from December 1847, maintained and published detailed notes of his cases. He preferred chloroform to ether but recognised its greater power, and, unusually for the time, employed an assistant to supervise the anaesthesia.[59] Matters went less well in Berlin where the first chloroform to be administered was to a bear at the zoo, which was blinded by cataracts. The operation was a success but the bear did not regain consciousness, and its death from *Das Chloroform* was immortalised both in verse and a bronze sculpture.[60]

Inexorably, the use of chloroform spread throughout the continent of Europe, notably in Italy, Austria, Russia, and Scandinavia, while British surgeons took it to India. The situation was more complicated in the United States.

Chloroform was tried throughout the North-eastern states, and in February it was reported that 'Messrs W.B. Little and Co., Hanover Street, Boston, are manufacturing this new agent in large quantities. . . . The demand for chloroform almost exceeds belief',[61] but after this initial enthusiasm, the first reports of fatalities greatly restricted its use, and Boston in particular reverted to and remained faithful to ether. The Southern states, influenced by New Orleans, whose doctors had studied in Paris, followed the French fashion, and quickly changed their preference to chloroform, which was soon adopted across the rest of the USA and Canada, although it did not entirely replace ether, and the two were often combined in a mixture.

In November 1848, Simpson, with absolute confidence in both Scottish methods and the Scottish product, was able to write that in the last twelve months hardly an operation had been performed in Edinburgh without the use of chloroform.[62] There had been no deaths in Edinburgh, and he was happy to dismiss reports of deaths elsewhere as due to causes other than the anaesthetic, or even entirely fictitious. In London, which did not have the acclaim of priority, matters were given a more critical eye, though a new and influential champion was about to emerge. In January 1849 when Catherine, wife of Charles Dickens was about to give birth to her eighth child, her doctors were extremely reluctant to administer chloroform, and it was only given at her husband's insistence. 'I am convinced' Dickens wrote, after Catherine's pain-free delivery 'that it is as safe in its administration as it is miraculous in its effects.'[63] Dickens, a man of great enthusiasms, cannot have failed to communicate his beliefs to London society.

FOUR

UNDER THE INFLUENCE

> We know not, and cannot know, where safety ends, and danger begins, by any known action of the agent, or by any law of its action.
>
> *Walter Channing MD, 1848*[1]

Within a year of its introduction, chloroform was a worldwide phenomenon, and the anaesthetic of choice everywhere save the North-eastern United States. Its speedy action was a particular recommendation to surgeons who had not developed the confident, successful and surprisingly safe Boston method of 'pushing' an ether-soaked sponge on to a struggling patient. The profound, relaxed and extended degree of unconsciousness produced by chloroform heralded a brave new era of surgery, in which delicate and lengthy procedures could maximise the preservation of healthy tissue.

Newspapers eagerly reported successful operations during which the patient felt no pain and afterwards expressed wonderment and gratitude. In January 1848, Thomas Wakley jnr, surgeon to the Royal Free Hospital and son of the editor of the *Lancet*, carried out an intricate dissecting out of bones from the ankle, the first operation of its kind, which took several painstaking minutes, and was keenly watched by an audience of medical men who were duly impressed.[2] In Liverpool a twelve-year-old girl, who had suffered for four years with a diseased knee, had her leg amputated, after which she was reported to have 'looked calmly around her and asked "Oh! Is it off?"'.[3] The *Liverpool Chronicle* commented, 'The utility of this new discovery needs no further eulogies. . . .' In 1848 Dr John Hancorn published a pamphlet called *Observations on Chloroform in Parturition* designed to encourage nervous patients. 'I never had so good a time; it was very quick,' he reported one lady as saying, '. . . well it's a very good thing, Mr Hancorn, a very good thing, and if I was about to be confined again tomorrow, I should wish to have it, and I will tell any one so.'[4] There were numerous testimonials in a similar vein, suggesting that the most powerful and rapid method by which the news was spread may well have been word of mouth. As early as 15 January 1848 chloroform was sufficiently in the public arena that a report of an acrimonious debate at the Liverpool town council at which a Mr Holme and a Mr Evans traded stinging insults, drew the comment, 'Some persons uncharitably believe that by way of deadening pain, Mr Samuel Holme inhales the new chemical agency, chloroform, on these gala occasions.'[5]

Occasionally there were those who claimed that they could not be chloroformed. Simpson believed that this was because when they awoke they were able to pick up the thread of the preceding conversation at once, and were not aware of any pause. One student presented himself for an experiment to prove his point. He soon went under, and Simpson decided to demonstrate that his subject had been anaesthetised by removing his shoes and socks before he awoke. The young man, who prided himself on being something of a dandy, woke up to find he was revealing some extremely dirty feet to the interested onlookers.[6] Another student who boasted a similar immunity was visited by friends in his lodgings, where he was given a good dose of chloroform, stripped naked, and laid out arrayed in a clean collar and cravat. They then rang for his landlady.[7]

Amidst all the euphoria there were some notable words of caution. Thomas Wakley jnr was particularly concerned that there might be some medical conditions which would render a patient unsuitable for anaesthesia. Early in 1848 he conducted a series of experiments on animals, showing that when they succumbed to the chloroform, the post-mortem revealed engorgement of the lungs and aneurism.[8] He advised that any patient with heart or lung disease should avoid both ether and chloroform, but thought the latter was the more dangerous. As the use of chloroform spread without harmful result, his advice was ignored.

There was, from a small, vociferous and influential minority, outright opposition, although this mainly related to minor surgery and midwifery, where it could be argued that the risks outweighed the benefits. Patients, too, had an instinctive nervousness about the concept of being rendered artificially unconscious. This rarely led to them refusing anaesthesia, rather it meant that they met it in a state of dread. Dreamy narcosis was one thing, but for some, the concept of a death-like sleep held dark terrors.

Flourens was initially of the opinion that chloroform did not deaden pain at all; in fact, he believed that the patient felt the pain even more strongly, but simply retained no memory of it afterwards. 'If we told our patients the truth,' he hinted ominously, 'it is probable that not one of them would wish to have an operation performed under chloroform, whereas they all insist on its use now because we shroud the truth in silence.'[9] Flourens was also concerned at the 'serious risk' that the use of chloroform might encourage surgeons to carry out more complex surgical procedures, in which humans would be living guinea-pigs.

Patients, in their ignorance, might have been eager to free themselves from the agonies of surgery, but many doctors, undeterred by a lack of supporting evidence, declared authoritatively that pain was not only useful but necessary to the proceedings, in that it actively prepared damaged tissues for repair. If this was true in surgery it was certainly true in midwifery. 'Pain,' trumpeted Dr Pickford, 'is the mother's safety, its absence her destruction.'[10]

Simpson, the great discoverer and promoter, at once took on the role as the champion of chloroform, and would spend the rest of his life fighting his corner with both fists, and blinkers firmly in place. Dismissing these arguments as 'aught else than indications of a strange degree of eccentricity of thought', he warned that decisions should be founded not on preconceptions, but factual evidence.[11] Simpson presented statistics collected from his own cases, showing that amputations were less likely to be fatal with than without an anaesthetic, and that maternal mortality increased with length of labour. Simpson, who could make unsupported sweeping statements as well as the next man, was impatient to the point of exasperation with those who did not share his ideas. His comments were often interpreted as a direct attack on the professional competence of his opponent, a reaction that he always greeted with some surprise.

Dr Robert Barnes, a London lecturer in midwifery, demanded to know what experiments had been carried out on animals that justified chloroform's use on human mothers. Recognising that Simpson's statistics on long labours did not prove that death was necessarily related to pain, while those on amputations had no relevance to childbirth, he criticised him for 'false analogy, bad arithmetic, and statistics run wild; however conclusive they may be to the judgement, and agreeable to the taste of the Edinburgh professor of midwifery'.[12]

Not only was pain good for the patient, it emerged, it was good for the surgeon, too. Surgeons who had once prided themselves on amputating a leg in less than a minute now protested that the patient's expressions of pain were an essential diagnostic tool. In labour, pain was a valuable guide to progress (Dr Barnes in particular described how he could judge the stages of labour by the kinds of moaning noises the patient made), and obstetricians protested that they relied on the mother's reactions when guiding their forceps. Simpson's reply was that they should know her anatomy better.

One lifelong critic of anaesthesia was the eminent Dr Charles Delucina Meigs, of Philadelphia. Meigs, born in 1792, was appointed to the chair of obstetrics at Jefferson Medical College in 1843. Of strong personality and undoubted skill and authority, he regarded labour pains as 'a most desirable salutary and conservative manifestation of the life force'.[13] One of his chief objections to chloroform was that he believed its effects to be no different from drunkenness, which, it went without saying, was a bad thing. Meigs once said that a woman 'has a head almost too small for intellect and just big enough for love',[14] and maybe this is the secret of why he did not take female agonies seriously. Simpson, in contrast, was ahead of his time, and certainly of Meigs, in his attitude towards women's intellect, which extended to his approval of their entry into the medical profession; and he later employed Emily Blackwell, sister of a pioneer woman doctor, as an assistant.

Where Simpson was confident, sometimes to the point of foolhardiness, Meigs exemplified caution. He did make the wholly reasonable point that the effects of anaesthetics on the brain were as yet unknown, a matter to which it seems Simpson had given no thought at all. He also, like many others, suggested that anaesthesia could suspend the contractions of the uterus, though no one had any means of measuring either the dose of anaesthetic the patient was receiving or the strength of contractions. In the end, that controversy was stilled by the plain evidence that thousands of women were defying medical opinion by successfully giving birth under anaesthesia.

Chloroform naturally fell under suspicion whenever a death occurred after its use, and there were fears that anaesthesia was responsible for complications such as haemorrhage, convulsions, paralysis, pneumonia, inflammation and mental derangement in the patient, and idiocy, hydrocephalus, and convulsions in the newborn. Dr Paton of Dundee told Simpson of two cases where ladies had died of puerperal fever, and the public had attributed it to the chloroform since when it had been difficult to overcome the prejudice.[15] Time bore out Simpson's denials that chloroform was responsible for any of these complications and, indeed, chloroform was later used as a treatment for convulsions.

Simpson's prediction that patients themselves would force the use of chloroform upon their doctors was, in the event, quite correct, but it was not what doctors wanted to hear or how they thought they should act. Many were outraged at the suggestion that they might be dictated to by their patients. The public were important allies for Simpson, especially women, who begged for relief from their labour pains. Many a nervous and reluctant doctor, with little knowledge and no training, found himself applying the chloroformed handkerchief. Simpson's promotion of chloroform as delicious and easy to use suggested that even the lay public could safely employ it. Lord Blantyre wrote to him in December 1847 wanting some to keep in his house in case of a bad accident, plus a supply for the village doctor, and asked to be sent two bottles of a pint each with directions for use.[16]

There were a few objections from women. Some religious souls felt guilty, though this was usually after they had relieved the agonies of childbirth. There were also a few women past childbearing years who wore their past suffering like a badge and initially begrudged the fact that their daughters were to be spared pain, though after the event they were inevitably grateful.

EROTIC DREAMS

There was another unlooked-for aspect of anaesthesia that caused severe difficulty to Victorian sensibilities – its power as a sexual stimulant. The idea that women in labour might experience erotic dreams was considered by some to be reason enough to withhold pain relief. The most persistent exponent of that view was Dr George Thompson Gream, of Queen Charlotte's Lying-in Hospital, whose attempts at a high moral tone only served to make him ridiculous. Gream (a married man who never became a father) seized upon a paper contributed to the *Lancet* by a Dr Tyler Smith in 1847, referring to a case where a young Frenchwoman, giving birth to her second child, later confessed that under the influence of ether she had dreamed of having sexual intercourse with her husband. 'To the women of this country the bare possibility of having feelings of such a kind excited and manifested in outward uncontrollable actions would be more shocking even to anticipate than the endurance of the last extremity of physical pain,' claimed Smith.[17]

Gream theorised that a person under ether or chloroform would dream of any part of the body that was irritated, so the pressure of the foetal head would cause sexual dreams. In the case described by Smith, he revealed, the young woman in labour had actually offered to kiss the male attendant. The idea of this happening to a modest young woman he found revolting. If women could only be made aware of this, 'they would undergo even the most excruciating torture, or I believe, suffer death itself, before they would subject themselves to the shadow of a chance of exhibitions such as have been recorded'.[18] With a strong sense of delicacy, he added: 'The facts . . . are unfit for publication in a pamphlet that may fall into the hands of persons not belonging to the medical profession.'[19]

Gream stated authoritatively and despite overwhelming evidence to the contrary that everyone else was rapidly coming around to his way of thinking, and that anaesthesia in normal childbirth would soon become a thing of the past. Women of rank and education in society had, according to Gream, an aversion to the use of chloroform, and were willing to endure the pain. He distributed a circular letter to medical men, asking for examples of cases where chloroform had caused harm to the patient, and in a second pamphlet published in 1849 claimed that their responses exceeded even his fears. There was no lack of evidence in both published reports and correspondence that patients experienced sexual excitement under chloroform. Most of these cases concerned women, but Gream quoted two cases of men being treated for stricture of the urethra who afterwards could only with difficulty be convinced that there had not been any females in the room.

Gream's obsession with sex, and his harping on the subject at professional meetings, ensured that the perfectly reasonable concerns about safety which formed the bulk of his writing were lost in the howls of derision at what appeared to be his obvious arousal thinly disguised by an assumed virtue. Matters were not helped by his deliberate distortion of facts and statistics to support his views.

Simpson attacked without mercy, saying that the allegations had been 'repeated and gloated over by those who have propounded it in a way which forms, apparently unconsciously on their own part, the severest self-inflicted censure upon the sensuality of their own thoughts'. The writer was not 'entitled to imagine that his own lewd thoughts are typified in the thoughts or actions of his patients'.[20] He added firmly that he had never seen the behaviour described by Gream, and neither had any of his colleagues. In Simpson's retelling of the case quoted by Tyler Smith, the Frenchwoman and her husband were transformed into a prostitute and her lover, and clearly a French prostitute could have nothing in common with an English lady. Gream's regular attendance at meetings of the Westminster Surgical Society ensured that the subject continued to be debated for another two years, much to the weariness and irritation of the other members. At one such meeting he referred to cases where women under the influence of chloroform had used obscene and disgusting language, which he believed was in itself sufficient argument that chloroform should never be used by English women.[21] A Dr Rogers must surely have been deriding Gream when he retorted that in *his* practice patients under the influence of chloroform 'prayed eloquently and had sung psalms and hymns in an angelic strain'![22]

Gream soon wisely fell silent, and returned to what must have promised to be a career of relative obscurity. That it was not ultimately so suggests that, despite his faults, Dr Gream must have been a highly capable obstetrician.

PUBLIC REACTION

Interest in chloroform was such that when in January 1848 William Brande, a chemistry professor, gave a lecture on ether and chloroform at the Royal Institution, there was a large and eager audience for his wisdom, not only of medical men, but the general public, including some ladies.[23] After discussing the composition of chloroform, and showing that it was not inflammable, Brande proposed to illustrate its safety in use by an experiment. A guinea-pig, a nonchalant veteran of earlier demonstrations, was placed under a glass dome on a sheet of absorbent paper, and a drachm of chloroform was introduced through a tube. For some minutes nothing appeared to happen, and Brande continued his talk. On previous occasions the guinea-pig had succumbed to the chloroform by keeling over on its side but on this occasion its legs simply buckled and it flopped down on its belly. It was some while before Brande realised that his subject was unconscious, and he quickly removed it from the dome, held it up to show that it was indeed asleep, and then placed it on one side to recover. Alas, the delay had proved fatal, and the guinea-pig had been a guinea-pig for the last time. A writer to the *Lancet* was concerned that this accident would cause some alarm, since 'numerous have been the triumphant (?) quotations of this experiment as a clear and indisputable proof of the extreme danger of this agent',[24] while the *Lady's Newspaper* warned its readers against the extended use of chloroform, and cited the unfortunate demonstration as 'a useful illustration of the necessity of caution in using chloroform'.[25]

ENGLAND VERSUS SCOTLAND

Central to all debate and practices relating to chloroform for more than fifty years after its first use was the rapid polarisation of two conflicting schools of thought that disputed both its action and its correct mode of administration. A not unhealthy rivalry between English and Scottish medicine soon developed into a kind of trench warfare, with both sides deeply dug in, both sure that they were correct, and with deep animosity not to say contempt towards the other, losing no opportunity to lob verbal missiles or blow derisive raspberries. There was the Edinburgh school, personified by Simpson and James Syme, and the London school, whose leaders were John Snow and, later, Joseph Clover.

No one could have been more different from the passionate, larger-than-life Simpson than the stern and humourless surgeon James Syme. He was one of Simpson's bitterest critics, and had voted against him in the professorship election of 1839. The antipathy was mutual and the two men once quarrelled openly in a patient's house. Simpson, who believed that unflattering comments Syme had published about the role of accoucheurs were a personal attack, accused him to his face of improper and unprofessional conduct, while Syme, shaking with rage, countered with a similar accusation. Simpson later wrote to the president of the Royal College of Physicians about Syme's 'paroxysmal attacks on members of the profession' and his 'morbid appetite for professional controversy and railing'.[26]

Syme was a small, narrowly built man, with a lugubrious expression and a slight stutter in his speech. It was said of him that he never wasted a word, a drop of ink or a drop of blood. Born in 1799, he advanced through hard work rather than intellectual brilliance, but achieved some fame by the boldness with which he undertook dangerous and complex operations. He was appointed professor of surgery at Edinburgh University in 1833. At a time when many surgeons performed the most basic of amputations, cutting away the good with the bad, Syme believed in conservation. He developed many new techniques, including an amputation at the ankle that preserved the heel pad. Syme had firm ideas about the difference between his role and that of the Professor of Midwifery, and often resented what he saw as Simpson's intrusion into fields that were not appropriate to him. His pre-eminence as a surgeon gave him a confidence in his own methods that amounted to arrogance, and he often ignored medical advances made by others to the great detriment of surgical practice in Scotland. What he had done he believed no one could improve upon. On one matter, however, Simpson and Syme were in agreement, and that was on the use of chloroform. Syme began by opposing it, but was rapidly converted, not only to its use, but to Simpson's method, for which he gave him full credit, and on which he treated students to a ten-minute lecture. Syme, although without Simpson's obvious charisma, was nevertheless considered to be an excellent teacher. He exerted a prodigious influence on both his students and assistants, who idolised him and preached his doctrines long after his death, an endurance of ideas that later had a profound impact on the history of chloroform.

In Edinburgh, every medical student, after a brief grounding in the principles of anaesthesia, was expected to take turns in administering chloroform for operations, using a fixed set of rules to which he was to adhere absolutely. The patient was to be horizontal, and the method of administration, the handkerchief. Inhalers were dismissed as useless at best, dangerous at worst. Dose was irrelevant, as was any consideration of the individual patient's fitness to receive chloroform. The administrator was to monitor respiration, and attention to the pulse was considered to be not only unnecessary, but a dangerous distraction. Syme did recognise that stertorous breathing was a serious matter, and advised that when this occurred the tongue should be seized with a pair of artery forceps and pulled well forward. These rules were sufficiently rigid that if there was any condition which might make anaesthesia difficult, for example in an operation on the mouth or jaw, then it was simply not used at all. As late as 1864 Syme removed a cancerous tongue without any anaesthetic, for fear the patient would choke on the blood, a problem which other surgeons had solved fourteen years before. In English schools, while there were lectures and demonstrations, students were given far less or even no practical experience. Simply put, in Edinburgh, where anyone could anaesthetise, everyone did, but in London where it was a complex matter, the move was towards the specialist anaesthetist.

London doctors followed the advice of John Snow, who was obsessed by the kind of meticulous measurement that Edinburgh men regarded with amused contempt. He was convinced that an instrument was essential to regulate the percentage of chloroform in the inhaled air, and his initial findings suggested that the concentration of chloroform in air should not exceed 5 per cent. He saw no dangers in having the patient seated in a comfortable easy chair where appropriate, and advised monitoring of both respiration and pulse, the pulse being more important.

Inspired by Snow, English doctors were busy devising new chloroform inhalers. Many were simple face-masks of cloth, wickerwork or perforated metal, with a space to hold a chloroform-soaked sponge, while the more solid ones had separate valves to admit air and carry away exhalations. Protheroe Smith, a London obstetrician who claimed to be the first to use ether in England, devised a graduated jar, which allowed for inspired air to be drawn through a reservoir of chloroform, rather after the manner of a hookah. Snow's inhaler was far more complex. The face-piece was of thin sheet lead, which could be moulded to the patient's features, while a valve enabled atmospheric air to be admitted. A tube connected the face-piece to a structure of three nested cylinders. As the patient inhaled, air was drawn into the space between the second and inner cylinder, passing over a coil of absorbent paper saturated in chloroform, then passing up the inner cylinder to the breathing tube. The space between the second and outer cylinder was filled with cold water, to create a constant level of evaporation. Not all English practitioners used inhalers. St Bartholomew's Hospital preferred a simple oval sponge, covered in oilskin, its hollow shape ensuring that the liquid did not touch the face. General practitioners, who applied chloroform to patients in their own homes, found that special apparatus was an expensive and cumbersome option and they preferred the simplicity of a handkerchief or towel.

There was one matter, however, that both camps appeared to be agreed upon – the only danger in chloroform administration was accidental overdose, and this could be easily avoided by ensuring a free supply of air. The only external sources of risk to the patient were therefore bad chloroform and medical incompetence. The first chloroform deaths were to provoke a long and bitter controversy.

DEATH IN NEWCASTLE

Hannah Greener, of Winlaton in Newcastle upon Tyne, had had an unfortunate start in life. She was illegitimate, and her mother had died when she was born. Her general health was good, but a persistent problem of ingrowing toenails caused her a great deal of pain. In January 1848 it was apparent to the family physician, Dr Meggison, that the nail on the right big toe would have to be removed. A few months previously she had had a toenail removed from her left foot under ether at the Infirmary, after which she had been unwell. Meggison therefore decided to use chloroform, which he had every reason to believe was both easier and safer.

On Friday 28 January, Hannah spent the morning fretting nervously at the prospect of the operation, though this did not prevent her from fortifying herself with a large meal. When Meggison and his assistant, Mr Lloyd, arrived at the house at one o'clock, she at once burst into tears. The sobbing girl was seated in an armchair in front of a warm fire, while Mr Lloyd laid out his instruments. Meggison tapped her on the shoulder, and told her to give over crying as she would soon be better. The only other person present was John Rayne, her uncle.

Meggison had given chloroform many times before, and determined that only a very small amount would be required for such a minor operation, which was hardly likely to take more than a minute. He poured a teaspoonful on to a pocket-handkerchief, and gently brought it to the girl's face, keeping it moving and allowing sufficient distance to ensure an adequate supply of air, while Mr Lloyd monitored the patient's pulse, and Rayne steadied Hannah's leg. After two breaths Hannah found something objectionable in it, or perhaps her nerves got the better of her, for she pulled the doctor's hand away, but he persuaded her to place her hands on her knees and breathe naturally. The inhalation resumed for about half a minute after which her eyes closed. Breathing and pulse remained normal, the rigidity of her arm muscles suggesting that anaesthesia had been produced. Meggison withdrew the handkerchief, and after examining a pupil and pinching a cheek, instructed Lloyd to proceed with the operation. At the first incision, the girl gave a small convulsive jerk, which led Meggison to believe that she was not sufficiently under, and he began to apply more chloroform to the handkerchief.

Hannah's breathing had seemed stronger and faster since the cloth had been removed, then, to everyone's surprise, it suddenly became very rapid. Abruptly, her face and lips became blanched, then there was a moan, a splutter, one or two weak breaths, and finally, nothing. Meggison dropped the handkerchief, called for cold water, and dashed it in her face, then tried to get her to drink some. He called for brandy, and attempted to trickle some down her throat, but she was unresponsive, though he thought she might have swallowed some. He raised her eyelids and they remained open, showing that her eyes were bloodshot. By now thoroughly alarmed, and fearing the worst, Meggison laid the patient upon the ground and tried to bleed her, first from the arm, then the jugular. Barely a spoonful of blood oozed out. Hannah Greener was dead. From the first inspiration of chloroform to this horrible conclusion had taken scarcely two minutes.

Two men were called in for the post-mortem, eminent Newcastle surgeon Sir John Fife, and Dr Robert Mortimer Glover of Newcastle Medical School, the latter being the same gentlemen who had conducted the animal experiments in 1842, and who may well still have been smarting with indignation at Simpson's rebuff. The most obvious internal symptom concerned the lungs, which they found 'in a very high state of congestion'. Fife was confident that this was the cause of death, produced by the inhalation of chloroform, and the jury agreed. No blame was attached to anyone, since Fife declared that he had every confidence in chloroform, and attributed its fatal effect to a 'peculiarity in the constitution of the young woman'. Although Fife had described Hannah as 'a well-grown girl' he had also stated that she was thin, which led many of those commenting on the case to conclude incorrectly that she was in feeble health.[27]

The verdict satisfied neither the Edinburgh nor the London schools. Snow had observed that residues of chloroform vapour in the lungs meant that its effects could continue to accumulate for up to twenty seconds after inhalation was discontinued, so it was the strength of the vapour and not the amount of liquid used which was critical. Even with one teaspoonful, he believed that the use of a handkerchief rather than an inhaler had led to Hannah Greener being overdosed. Simpson's view was that death was not due to chloroform at all, which was present in too low a dose to be dangerous. He declared that the girl had simply fainted, and if she had been left alone she would have recovered. He was confident that death was due to her choking on the water and brandy, a conclusion which not even the *Edinburgh Medical and Surgical Journal* could share with him. Dr Glover ridiculed Simpson's attempt to divert blame away from chloroform, and disagreed with Snow. He had conducted some experiments on dogs, in which some had been poisoned with chloroform and others drowned by being forcibly held under water, and observed that the post-mortem appearances in the lungs were different. The true cause of death in the Greener case was, he believed, chloroform syncope.[28] The expression 'chloroform syncope', meaning loss of consciousness caused by the action of chloroform on the heart, was destined to appear very frequently in the medical press, and be another cause of fierce contention between the English and Scottish schools.

It would be almost 50 years before physiologists began to understand how Hannah Greener had died, and these were years of debate, research, argument, frustration and rage. In the meantime, everyone resolved to be a little more careful, happy that apart from the occasional idiosyncratic and therefore unpredictable reaction, all would be well. All was not well. Hannah Greener's was only the first of thousands of unexplainable deaths which Sir James Simpson was able to convince himself were not caused by chloroform.

A SOURCE OF IRRITATION

Early in 1848 a physician in the south of England complained to Simpson that chloroform was too great an irritant to inhale, and it caused coughing and bronchitis. Simpson at once obtained a supply from a London manufacturing house. He too found it highly irritant, and on testing it with litmus paper, found it was emitting acidic fumes, which he identified as hydrochloric acid. Simpson knew that chloroform was said to decompose, but denied that this ever happened with Scottish chloroform, saying that the London product was greatly inferior as it contained impurities.

The high quality of Edinburgh chloroform became one of the cornerstones of the Scottish 'method'. Many manufacturers used the process advised by William Gregory, a professor of chemistry who issued his own personal certificates of purity to those who met with his approval. In 1850 Gregory's approved chloroform developed suffocating odours and a greenish deposit, and had to be recalled at considerable loss.[29] Even Duncan and Flockhart were not exempt. In 1851 a sample of their finest chloroform was placed on display at the Great Exhibition, and decomposed overnight.[30] Pharmacists blamed a fault in the manufacturing process, though what this was they couldn't say.

There was an eager seeking after purity by doctors on both sides of the Tweed, many of whom wrote to the *Lancet* suggesting tests to assure themselves of the scrupulous perfection of their chloroform, and describing methods of washing it clean of such nasty contaminants as alcohol. Failure in this essential was stated to be the cause of blistering of the patient's lips, vomiting after surgery, and death. It would be a number of years before it was finally accepted that pure chloroform did indeed decompose in daylight, that alcohol was a preservative, and that hydrochloric acid was the least of the problems.

FIVE

HER MAJESTY IS A MODEL PATIENT

Dr Snow gave that blessed chloroform and the effect was soothing, quieting and delightful beyond measure.

Queen Victoria[1]

The regular meetings of the Westminster Medical Society were a good place for an aspiring young doctor to make his mark. Matters of current importance were actively debated, papers were presented, and anyone, irrespective of status, was entitled to listen and speak. In 1837 a timid young medical student from the north of England joined the society. Thin and ascetic, his high forehead accentuated by an incipiently receding hairline, his voice was quiet and husky. Though he spoke well, and to the point, he at first made little impression. Only gradually did it become apparent to the other members that his was no ordinary mind and that they would do well to give him their attention. His name, they noted, was John Snow. Knowledgeable, calm and meticulous, he had all the necessary qualities to carry out a highly sensitive task – giving chloroform to Queen Victoria.

Snow was born in York on 15 March 1813, the eldest of nine children. His father, William, was at that time a labourer, though in later years he was able to purchase land and became a farmer. Lack of funds did not seem to be an impediment to young John's education and it is probable that he received some financial assistance from his mother's brother, Charles Empson, a much-travelled man of some means. After private schooling, Snow went to Newcastle upon Tyne to be apprenticed to a Dr William Hardcastle. He was there for six years and during this time became convinced of the advantages of vegetarianism, and also became a teetotaller and an active member of the temperance movement.

After two more short apprenticeships, Snow arrived in London in 1836 to study at the Hunterian School of Medicine, and later practised at the Westminster Hospital. He completed his studies in 1838, when he took humble rooms in Frith Street, Soho, and commenced as a general practitioner. He lived simply, ate frugally, dressed plainly, and kept little company apart from his science books. Those who knew him professionally thought him very quiet and reserved in his manner, and perhaps a little strange, though undoubtedly very clever.

He took an early interest in both respiration and the use of instruments, and the first paper he presented to the Westminster Medical Society was on the subject of asphyxia and the resuscitation of newborn children. In this he described a mechanism that could inflate the lungs and carry away expired air. More papers followed, which were well received. He was working so hard that it was not until December 1844 that he took and passed his MD examination at London University.

As a young man Snow's health had been good and he had been noted as a strong swimmer, but in 1844 he suffered from what was then known as *phthisis pulmonaris*, or tuberculosis of the lungs. His treatment was to spend a lot of time in the fresh air, and he appears to have recovered. In the following year he suffered severe kidney disease, and was advised to relax from his strict vegetarian diet and take a little wine, which he did. His health improved, but before long he had embarked on the same course as Simpson, that of self-experimentation with a variety of dangerous vapours.

Dr Snow had still not met with any great success in his profession when, at thirty-four, he took an interest in the new art of etherisation. He saw that it was still regarded with some caution, which he attributed to the lack of an effective inhaler, and set about designing an improved model, carrying out experiments on animals and himself. While many of his animal experiments necessarily and deliberately ended in the death of the subject, he always took care to minimise suffering.

One day he happened to bump into a druggist he knew, hurrying along with a large ether apparatus under his arm. He greeted the friend, who was disinclined to stop and talk, as he said he was 'giving ether here and there and everywhere, and am getting quite into an ether practice'.[2] Snow was well aware that the man had no idea of the physiology involved in this work, and thought that if such a man could get a bustling ether practice, perhaps some scraps of the same thing might fall to him. Accordingly, Snow went to St George's Hospital with his own ether inhaler, and asked to be allowed to anaesthetise the dental patients. A Dr Fuller saw his work and was sufficiently impressed to recommend him to a surgeon. He soon came to the notice of the eminent London surgeon Robert Liston, and before long was accepted as the leading ether man in London. His extensive experience, backed up by meticulous notes and experimental work aimed at a full understanding of his field, earned him considerable respect. The quiet man was now a name. Success and a comfortable income were usually the precursors to matrimony, yet this always eluded the reserved Dr Snow, whose name was never linked romantically to another. It was one of the regrets of his life, especially as he professed to be very fond of children.

He made few close friends, but those few held him in great regard. After his death a Dr Attree wrote of him: 'Who does not remember his frankness, his cordiality, his honesty, the absence of all disguise or affectation under an apparent off-hand manner?' The Queen had lost a 'trustworthy, well-deserving, much esteemed subject'. The poor, to whom he often gave his services for nothing, had 'lost in him a real friend in the hour of need'.[3]

Personal pleasures, of which there were few, were never allowed to stand in the way of Snow's dedication to his work. He was the personification of order, keeping a diary of every case in which he administered an anaesthetic, and detailed notes of his experiments. In his general practice he earned a reputation for sound judgement in diagnosis. He spent much of his time alone, but when in company, he had a pleasant, cheerful nature. His friend and biographer, Benjamin (later Sir Benjamin) Ward Richardson, found him 'full of humorous anecdotes', and while he did not read novels, which he felt were a waste of time, he enjoyed being read the more amusing character sketches of Dickens or Thackeray.

No sooner had Snow published the results of his work on ether than a new star appeared on the horizon, and ether was eclipsed. Recognising the advantages of chloroform, Snow dedicated himself to discovering its effects on the human system, and the best mode of applying it. Unlike the French physiologists, who then believed that anaesthesia was effectively asphyxia, Snow declared that it was more similar to narcosis. He did not then and never did believe that there was any disease or condition of general health that forbade the inhalation of either ether or chloroform. Even if there was disease of the heart or lungs he believed that the pain of an operation or the anticipatory fear was more harmful to the patient than the chloroform. He was not impressed by Wakley's experiments on animals, arguing that if a condition is found in death it does not necessarily mean it is present in life. He realised that the lung congestion found by Wakley was caused by the circulation continuing briefly after respiration had ceased.

While Scottish doctors were dismissing the necessity of measuring chloroform at all, Snow believed that safety depended on regulating the percentage of chloroform vapour in inspired air, which could only be achieved with an apparatus. Initially, he advised 5 per cent as a maximum. He was also aware that air temperature affected the amount of chloroform that vaporised. Thus his inhaler was encased in a water bath, the water never to exceed the temperature of 60°F. The exuberant tone of Simpson's pamphlet had led many doctors to believe that chloroform was safer than ether, but Snow's experiments revealed that chloroform was much the more powerful agent, and he knew that care was essential. He deplored Simpson's instructions to apply one or two teaspoonfuls rapidly on a handkerchief, and was offended by the careless enthusiasm of Professor Miller, who believed that apparatus was dangerous and advised the use of any handy absorbent material, saying that on occasions even a nightcap or the glove of an onlooker had been pressed into service.[4]

In natural labour Snow advocated light anaesthesia, which would not affect the uterus or the child. In such cases, where the dose was very small, he did not disdain the use of a handkerchief. He had observed that infants born of chloroformed mothers did not, in the first minute of life, kick and scream with quite the same vigour as those whose mothers had not been anaesthetised, but did not think that this was harmful.[5]

Snow recognised and described five different stages of the effects produced by chloroform. In the first, there was some exhilaration, and decreased sensibility, although the patient remained conscious. In the second, mental functions were impaired; the patient was in a dreamy state, could hear what was said and could feel some pain. This was the stage he preferred for normal labour. In the third there were no voluntary motions, mental functions were abolished, and rigidity or spasms of the muscles could occur. The patient felt no pain, and it was in this stage that surgery could be carried out. In the fourth stage there was stertorous breathing, dilated pupils, and relaxed muscles. Snow considered that it was rarely necessary to go this far except in extreme cases of dislocations in muscular patients, during surgery near important vessels or in hard-drinking persons who were hard to keep quiet. In the fifth stage, which had been demonstrated in animal experiments, breathing became difficult due to paralysis of the chest muscles, and if the dose was continued, breathing would stop while the heart would continue pumping until arrested by asphyxia. He also commented, 'Those persons whose mental faculties are most cultivated appear usually to retain their consciousness longest whilst inhaling chloroform; and on the other hand, certain navigators and other labourers . . . having the smallest amount of intelligence, often lose their consciousness, and get into a riotous drunken condition, almost as soon as they have begun to inhale. There is a widely different class of person who also yield up their consciousness very readily, and get very soon into a dreaming condition when inhaling chloroform. I allude to hysterical females.'[6]

For children, natural labour, tooth-drawing and minor operations he thought it would be better to use something less powerful than chloroform. His experiments on animals had shown that ether could not produce paralysis of the heart; nevertheless, he continued to use chloroform, and on being asked why, said, 'I use chloroform for the same reason that you use phosphorus matches instead of the tinder box. An occasional risk never stands in the way of ready applicability.'[7]

Snow was the first person to recognise and measure the fact that the difference between an anaesthetic and a fatal dose of chloroform is extremely small. He calculated that to produce the third degree of anaesthesia it was necessary to absorb 18 minims of chloroform, for the fourth degree 24 minims was required, while 36 minims would arrest respiration. A minim is just one-sixtieth of a teaspoonful. He thus had a healthy respect for the powers of chloroform which was lacking in many of his contemporaries. Snow knew that if large doses were applied on a handkerchief, the doctor could not know how much the patient was receiving, and there was a risk of giving a dangerously high concentration.

Unlike many doctors, Snow was familiar with the work of Dumas, was well aware of the chemistry of chloroform, and knew that it would decompose in daylight. While Scottish doctors were attributing vomiting to impure English chloroform, Snow recognised very early the importance of restricting the amount of food in the stomach prior to surgery. Keenly aware of the power of Simpson's opinions, Snow dared to criticise the Scottish methods, and even declared that because of Simpson's influence, the practice of anaesthesia was in a less satisfactory state than if chloroform had never been introduced. When the first chloroform deaths occurred, which were ignored or dismissed by the Edinburgh school, it was to John Snow that London surgeons looked for an explanation.

Snow's reaction to the death of Hannah Greener was that she had suffered an overdose due to the administration of the chloroform on a handkerchief. He noted the circumstances carefully, so that when further surgical deaths occurred he was able to compare them. He didn't have long to wait. In February, a Mrs Simmons, of Cincinnati, aged thirty-five, expired after inhaling chloroform for a tooth extraction. The dentists had used an inhaler containing a chloroform-saturated sponge. In May, a thirty-year-old Boulogne woman required an operation to open an abscess. As in Hannah Greener's case, just one drachm of chloroform moistened a handkerchief, and like Hannah, she died without warning. Artificial respiration was tried with bellows; ammonia, cold air and cold water were applied, but to no avail. She was a plump lady and the post-mortem showed that her heart was flabby and loaded with fat while her stomach was full of food. The conclusion was that she had died from the effect of chloroform on an abnormal heart. It soon became an article of faith with doctors that 'fatty degeneration of the heart', something they could not predict, was the cause of death under chloroform. The French Academy later decided that this death was not due to chloroform but advised that being 'one of the most energetic agents' it was not to be used by inexperienced hands, and should never be used where there were contra-indications, or after meals.[8]

On 30 June 1848, plump, healthy-looking 22-year-old Walter Badger arrived at the surgery of Mr Robinson in Gower Street. Robinson, noted for having performed the first operation in England under ether, had since turned to chloroform. Badger was somewhat nervous of the procedure, and complained after inhaling from the sponge that it was not strong enough, so Robinson obligingly turned away to apply more chloroform. Badger was just commenting that the smell was very pleasant when without warning, his head fell forward and his arm dropped. Robinson splashed cold water on the patient, and tipped a pitcher of it over his head. A doctor was sent for who tried bleeding and artificial respiration without success. Mr Badger was dead. The post-mortem confirmed that Badger had a fat flabby heart, and an enlarged liver, and gave the cause of death as chloroform acting on these diseased organs. Snow did not attribute Badger's death to chloroform, as he had scarcely inhaled any, and stated 'it is probable that the immediate cause of death in this instance was fear'.[9]

In July, a letter was received from Hyderabad reporting that a timid and reluctant young woman requiring the amputation of a finger, had been given one drachm of chloroform on a handkerchief. She gave a little cough and after a few convulsive movements, died. In January 1849, in Lyons, a seventeen-year-old boy requiring amputation of a finger died under very similar circumstances, and in the same month the instant expiry was reported of a stout young man in Govan after inhaling chloroform for the removal of an ingrowing toenail. In February, Samuel Bennett, a 36-year-old mason's labourer, was due to have a big toe amputated. Half an ounce of chloroform failed to produce anaesthesia, and he had to wait two hours while fresh stocks were purchased. The second attempt was successful, and the toe was taken off, but when pressure was removed from the arteries, no blood flowed. Every attempt at artificial respiration failed.

Doctors were mystified. They had already noted an apparent anomaly that was going to puzzle and mislead them for many years to come. In animal experiments, it was the breathing that stopped first, but in humans, it appeared to be the heart. Snow had initially agreed with the Edinburgh school that breathing stopped before the pulse. However he later observed from his work on animals that the heart would stop first if chloroform was given in concentrations of 10 per cent or more. In the human deaths, however, the dose had apparently been very low. Snow surmised that despite appearances, the patients must have accidentally received a large concentration. In cases where it could not be denied that the patient had inhaled very little chloroform, he reasoned that death had to be due to something else, such as shock or fright.

Prior to the first chloroform deaths, if a surgeon had been asked to predict which patients would be the most susceptible, he would probably have cited children, the elderly, the feeble, and those undergoing the most severe operations. The pattern that was emerging was quite different. Those who succumbed were for the most part young, healthy, and muscular, were undergoing only minor medical procedures, and tended to struggle during the induction. Excessively nervous and agitated patients, like Hannah Greener, were also more likely to expire, as were alcoholics, and there were twice as many deaths among males than there were in the apparently frailer sex. It was a confusing array of clues, and no one really knew what to make of them. Snow later modified his conclusions. The young and healthy, he said, were more likely to struggle against the chloroform, and hold their breath. On the next inspiration, they took in too high a percentage. His answer was to insist on slow and gradual administration. Nevertheless, patients did occasionally die when his inhaler was used, which he suggested was due to incorrect adjustment of the absorbent paper.

The difficulty in arriving at cause of death was very understandable. Monitoring of a patient during anaesthesia was done by external observation. The action of chloroform was still a matter for theory and speculation, and doctors were severely hampered by the status of surgery at the time. The experience they had of seeing healthy organs in a living patient was extremely limited, and it was hard for them to draw conclusions from what they saw in post-mortems. In 1850 Dr Snow presented to the Westminster Medical Society an apparatus he had devised for detection of chloroform in a dead body. Vapour from the heated material was passed across silver nitrate and any chloroform would form a white precipitate of chloride of silver. It could detect one-hundredth of a grain in 1,000 grains of water, and he had already used it, having been supplied with some of the viscera of a woman found dead, concluding that her death was not due to chloroform.

Anatomist Francis Sibson often collaborated with Snow. Carefully analysing the first four deaths, he concluded that the cause was instant paralysis of the heart, and believed that the patient's fear made the administration of chloroform more dangerous.[10] Snow, who advised calming the patient before an operation to allow more tranquil breathing, believed it was impossible that a state of mind could combine with chloroform to cause danger, because an unconscious patient would feel no fear. Snow had personal experience of only one chloroform death – that of an elderly man in 1852, which he was able to satisfy himself was not due to the anaesthetic.

Where chloroform was most in favour, the deaths did little to affect its use. It was already obvious that in major surgery it saved lives, and while it was perhaps not as safe as had originally been thought, and the slapdash confidence had mellowed, it seemed that all that was required to make it safe was a little care in administration, and a prior examination of the patient for potential heart or lung disease. John Bennet writing in January 1850 stated, 'we cannot but admit its inhalation to be attended with a certain amount of risk. That this risk is very slight indeed, is proved by the very small number of fatal cases recorded. . . . I do not think that the fatal instances that have occurred imply such an amount of danger as to induce us to forgo the benefit of chloroform.'[11] At that time, little work had been done on the comparative risks of chloroform and ether, so doctors stayed with the one that was easier and pleasanter to use.

There were a few exceptions. In Lyons, senior surgeon J.E. Pétrequin, who had made an early trial of chloroform after reading favourable reports, was sufficiently alarmed by several sudden and unpredictable deaths that he at once returned to using ether, and started a campaign to encourage others to do the same. He was unsuccessful in France; indeed, he reported that by 1850 in Paris 'ether was almost forgotten; there was an exaggerated admiration for chloroform. . . . Nothing, in fact could disillusion their minds'.[12] This was particularly true of a Dr Sédillot of Strasbourg, who at a meeting of the Société de Chirurgie in Paris in October 1851 was adamant that chloroform 'properly administered, in a pure state, never kills'.[13] A visiting Italian surgeon influenced a return to ether in Naples, but on the whole, continental Europe remained faithful to chloroform for very many more years.

Things were different where there was greater expertise in the use of ether, and confidence in its superior safety. At the Massachusetts General Hospital, chloroform was banned within a very short time of its introduction. In the other Northern United States, chloroform lost favour, though it still had its adherents, who believed that it could be managed with caution.

The attitude in Edinburgh was epitomised by the comments of a Dr Skae who said: 'The successful employment of chloroform in surgery and obstetrics north of the Tweed excites a strong impression that our professional brethren in the south must either employ a very impure preparation of the medicine or be very much at fault in their mode of exhibiting it.'[14]

Syme pointed to the smaller numbers of deaths in Scotland, but Snow responded that taking into account the differences in population the death rates were about the same. It was, in any case, impossible to produce accurate figures for deaths in Scotland, since at the time there were no coroners' inquests there. In England, reporters were always in attendance at any interesting inquest, so English newspapers carried frequent accounts of deaths under chloroform. There was a common belief, expressed by correspondents to both journals and newspapers, that no one ever died of chloroform in Scotland, and this reinforced the confidence of Scottish surgeons in the Edinburgh method. Over the years, two more beliefs arose concerning the use of chloroform. The fact that children took it readily led many to think that it was both safe and especially suitable for children, and women in labour were said to have a special immunity. In 1855, Snow believed there had been no deaths in children under fifteen; the only exception, a German case, he attributed to another cause, while in midwifery the classic chloroform death remained practically unknown.

Snow, looking for a way of preventing overdose, was the first person to try and deliver a precisely measured concentration of vapour to the patient. He devised a wholly novel apparatus, which he presented to the Westminster Medical Society in May 1849. It consisted of a large balloon, with a capacity of 2,000 cubic inches, provided with a tap and connected to a face-piece with valves. A measured quantity of chloroform was introduced into the balloon, which was then inflated with air by bellows, thus enabling the operator to know the exact proportion of chloroform inhaled. Snow announced that 3 per cent of vapour in the air was enough to produce insensibility in two minutes, and being uniformly mixed with air also made the inspired vapour less pungent. He used this apparatus a number of times with success, but found that the balloon sometimes got in the way of the surgeon, and inflating it was troublesome. The apparatus never came into general use. 'It seemed necessary,' he observed, 'to sacrifice a little of absolute perfection to convenience.'[15]

While Snow experimented with safer methods of administration, the search for a better anaesthetic continued. Thomas Nunneley, a Leeds surgeon, tested over thirty compounds on animals. He approved of Dutch liquid, and was enthusiastic about the properties of coal gas, but dismissive of ethylene (which was introduced as an anaesthetic in the twentieth century), although he also described the effects of a mixture of alcohol, chloroform and ether, in the ratio 1:2:3. This was later called the ACE mixture, and enjoyed some considerable use. In Austria and Italy there were experiments with mixtures of ether and chloroform. A ratio of 1 part chloroform to 6 or 8 parts ether was known as the Vienna mixture. Unfortunately, no one really understood to what extent the two vapours actually mixed, and it was difficult to determine what the patient was actually receiving. In May 1848 a Dr Gabb wrote to the *Lancet* and suggested mixing ether and chloroform in the proportions two-thirds ether to one-third chloroform,[16] but a Dr Jones responded that he didn't think this was possible given their different specific gravities.[17] Gabb replied that in his experience they did mix, although he did not know if by so doing they formed another compound, an ignorance which didn't stop him from using the unknown vapour on his patients.[18]

Instead of a mixture, some surgeons advocated giving the two vapours serially, but there were differing opinions as to which should be given first. Induction was much swifter with chloroform, and the excitement and choking could be avoided, but on the other hand they were well aware that many of the deaths under chloroform occurred during the initial phase.

Although Snow became an acknowledged expert in the administration of chloroform he also continued the search for the perfect anaesthetic. He tested several gases, such as carbon dioxide, carbon monoxide, and nitrogen, as well as a number of volatile liquids, many of which are now known to be highly toxic. His first step was to ascertain their effects on animals, and if they seemed promising as possible anaesthetics, he then, despite the earnest and repeated pleas of his friends, experimented upon himself. The eight substances which he particularly concentrated on were chloroform, ether, the highly explosive ethyl nitrate, benzin and Dutch liquid, both of which had already been rejected by Simpson as intolerable, and three chemicals which are now recognised health hazards, bromoform, ethyl bromide, and carbon disulphide.

ANAESTHETIST TO THE QUEEN

In 1853 Queen Victoria was pregnant with her eighth child. By now Snow was regarded as one of the leading men in his field, and had moved the year before into more affluent lodgings in Sackville Street. Five years previously, before the birth of Princess Louise, it had been rumoured that Professor Simpson would be required to give the queen chloroform, but this had swiftly been denied. By 1850, however, it was clear that her majesty had been considering the matter, for when she was again due to give birth, discreet enquiries were made by the royal accoucheur, Sir Charles Locock, about the possibility of chloroform being employed, and the man he consulted was John Snow.

In the event, Prince Arthur was born without its aid. In January 1853 Dr Snow administered chloroform to Miss Kerr, one of the royal ladies-in-waiting who was having a tooth extracted, and no doubt she reported back on her experience.[19] The queen was now determined to have chloroform for the coming confinement, and the prince consort arranged an interview with Dr Snow.

When Snow went to court, he dressed himself carefully in a court suit complete with sword and flattened hat. As he started out, a friend's child saw him and threw up her hands exclaiming, 'Oh, isn't Dr Snow *pretty*, Mama!' The mere idea of this rather plain and balding man being regarded as pretty he thought to be so droll that he often repeated the anecdote.[20] Snow was impressed by the prince's intelligent interest in the sciences, and the prince must have been impressed with the quiet learning of the modest doctor, for at that interview it was decided that the queen would have chloroform.

Dr Snow's notebook for the day records his administration of chloroform to the queen on Tuesday 7 April.[21] Dr Locock had been sent for at 9 a.m. and a hour later, Snow had received a note from the queen's physician, Sir James Clark, asking him to go to the Palace. Snow was shown to an apartment near that of the queen, which he shared with Clark, the second accoucheur Dr Ferguson, and, when he was not at the queen's bedside, Dr

Locock, until a little after midday, when the first stage of labour was almost over. 'At twenty past twelve by a clock in the Queen's apartment,' he recorded, 'I commenced to give a little chloroform with each pain, by pouring about fifteen minims by measure on a folded handkerchief.' The application reduced the pains to a trifling measure, and between contractions 'there was complete ease'. At no time did the queen lose consciousness. Dr Locock, who may have been sceptical of the procedure, expressed the opinion that the chloroform retarded labour and prolonged the intervals between contractions. At thirteen minutes past one by the clock, Prince Leopold was born safely, the queen having inhaled chloroform over a period of 53 minutes. Very shortly afterwards the placenta was expelled, and the queen appeared very cheerful and well, expressing herself much gratified with the chloroform. On the following day, Queen Victoria wrote to her uncle, 'I can report most favourably of it myself, for I have never been better or stronger.'[22]

There was no public announcement about the use of chloroform in the queen's confinement, but the newspapers carried the official circular from Buckingham Palace, which listed those actually present at the birth – Prince Albert, Dr Locock, Dr Snow and Nurse Lilly. Anyone familiar with Snow's speciality would have had a strong suspicion of why he was there. The news eventually came to the ears of Thomas Wakley snr, editor of the *Lancet*. Wakley had always been opposed to the use of chloroform in natural labour and, appalled by the thought that it had been applied to the queen, made some enquiries, and wrote, 'We were not at all surprised to learn that in her late confinement the Queen was not rendered insensible by chloroform or any other anaesthetic agent. We state this with feelings of the highest satisfaction.'[23]

Of course, it was quite true that the queen had not been rendered unconscious, but his informant must have worded his reply very carefully, mischievously allowing Wakley to jump to the wrong conclusion. Wakley then went on to make the ridiculous suggestion that officious meddlers at court had led to the 'pretence' of administering chloroform: 'We have felt irresistibly impelled to make the foregoing observations, fearing the consequences of allowing such a rumour respecting a dangerous practice in one of our national palaces to pass unrefuted. Royal examples are followed with extraordinary readiness by a certain class of society in this country.'[24]

In due course it must have become apparent to Mr Wakley that he had been fooled, but no breath of the subject was allowed to grace the pages of the *Lancet* again. The practice of administering an anaesthetic for each labour pain rather than continuously was not new, but from that time it became known as '*anaesthésie à la reine*' (sic).

Snow's patients started plying him for details of the queen's accouchement, but all he would say was, 'Her Majesty is a model patient.'[25] On one occasion he was applying chloroform to a lady who refused to go on taking any more until he told her word for word what the queen had said when she was taking it. 'Her Majesty,' he replied, 'asked no questions until she had breathed very much longer than you have, and if you will only go on in loyal imitation I will tell you everything.' The lady was silenced, and continued to take the chloroform as directed. Soon she was unconscious, and when she awoke, Dr Snow had left.[26]

On 20 October 1853 Snow saw another notable patient in labour. She was in a poor state of health, with extensive cavities of the lungs, but despite this he was able to administer chloroform, for which she expressed great relief. She was the daughter of the Archbishop of Canterbury, and there could hardly have been a better patient to demonstrate the approval of the religious establishment for the use of chloroform.[27] Many doctors who had opposed the idea of chloroform in natural labour now found themselves in a difficult position, since it was not only fashionable but endorsed by royalty and the Church. Some now stated that the new mode of administration had disposed of their earlier antipathy. One such was Dr George Thompson Gream, who in 1853 published a small pamphlet favouring light use of chloroform, even in uncomplicated labour. For this purpose he recommended a glass phial containing a chloroform-soaked sponge, which the patient could hold to her nostrils. The *Lancet*, observing that Gream, having previously derided others, now wished to take all the credit for himself, dismissed his idea contemptuously as a 'scent bottle'. There were still some opponents, such as Dr Robert Lee, who at a meeting in December 1853 read a paper called 'An account of seventeen cases of parturition in which chloroform was inhaled with pernicious effects', dismissed chloroform '*à la reine*' as 'mere pretence' calculated to deceive the weak, ignorant and credulous, and declared that 'in sorrow shalt thou bring forth children' was an established law of nature. Championing the cause of chloroform at that meeting was none other than Dr Gream.[28] The embracing of chloroform was a crucial fillip to Gream's career. He was appointed royal accoucheur in 1864 and was present at the birth of the future King George V.

On 14 April 1857, Dr Snow was again called to the Palace for the birth of the queen's last child, Princess Beatrice. Labour started at 2 a.m., and between 9 and 10 a.m. Prince Albert administered a very little chloroform on a handkerchief at each contraction. Dr Locock gave powdered ergot to assist the contractions and an hour later, Snow began his administration of chloroform, using just 10 minims on a handkerchief folded into a cone. More ergot was given at noon, and the queen complained that the chloroform was insufficient to remove the pain, and asked for more. By 1 p.m. she was tiring, and said she could not push when asked, so the chloroform was left off for three or four pains, and a final effort expelled the head, a little chloroform being given as the head emerged. The *Lancet* reported the use of chloroform without criticism.[29]

Snow's detailed notes of his cases show that during his career he administered chloroform approximately 450 times a year. His expertise, from both clinical work and experiment, was a valuable guide to other doctors. He also collected and published details of chloroform deaths from all over the world. Snow pioneered the use of chloroform in operations of the mouth, and was the first person to induce endotracheal anaesthesia (administered by a tube in the windpipe) in an animal experiment.

In 1858, Dr Snow was completing a major work, *On Chloroform and Other Anaesthetics*, in which he detailed all his findings on the subject, discussed the deaths and described his own cases and experiments. On 9 June, while hard at work, he was seized with a stroke, and although he made a partial recovery, suffered a second stroke a few days later. He died on 16 June, aged forty-five. It was left to his friend, Benjamin Ward Richardson, to prepare his manuscript for publication.

There are several memorials to Dr Snow. His friends erected a handsome monument to him in Brompton Cemetery that was destroyed by a bomb in 1941 but has since been restored. A college of the University of Durham at Stockton-on-Tees is named after him, while in 1955 a public house in Soho on the corner of

Broadwick Street and Lexington Street was renamed the John Snow: this contains a great deal of commemorative material.

When Queen Victoria's eldest daughter Vicky, the wife of Frederick William of Prussia, was about to give birth to her first child in January 1859, Snow had been dead a little over six months. The queen sent over her own physician, Sir James Clark, and a bottle of chloroform. The princess went into labour on 26 January, with Clark and Dr Wegner, the court physician, in attendance, neither of whom was willing to risk using the chloroform. It was a difficult labour. Dr Eduard Martin, chief of obstetrics at the University of Berlin, arrived the next day, finding Vicky in great pain and distress, the doctors in despair, and the obituaries about to be written. His examination showed that the child was in the breech position, and he at once took over the management of the labour and full responsibility for the consequences. He ordered Sir James Clark to dose Vicky with chloroform, while the anxious Wegner stood by begging him not to give her too much. Two-thirds of a bottle of chloroform later, Martin was able to extract an apparently lifeless infant. It was several minutes before his attempts at resuscitation took effect and the future Kaiser Wilhelm II took his first breath. Queen Victoria later wrote to Frederick's mother, Princess Augusta, 'Vicky appears to feel quite as well and to recover herself just as quickly as I always did. What a blessing she had chloroform! Perhaps without it her strength would have suffered very much.'[30]

SIX

THE CURE FOR ALL ILLS

> Take of: treacle four ounces, tincture of opium four ounces, tincture of capsicum three ounces, chloroform four ounces, dilute hydrocyanic acid one ounce, sulphuric ether four ounces, essence of peppermint half an ounce. Mix.
>
> *Recipe for chlorodyne published by the* British Medical Journal, *1862*[1]

In an era when the causes of most common diseases were unknown, it was inevitable that chloroform would be pressed into use for any painful ailment – not always appropriately. In July 1852 Dr Hall of Southwark wrote an angry letter to the *Lancet*.[2] In the previous issue, Dr Henry Behrend of Liverpool had confidently reported that chloroform was a cure for gonorrhoea.[3] His original treatment was injections of pure chloroform into the urethras of his suffering patients, but when they found this too painful, he diluted it with twice its volume of mucilage (a thin watery gum). The injections were given up to three times a day, and Behrend claimed that apart from some temporary pain, 'No evil effects have resulted from the application of the chloroform to the diseased portion of the urethra', and described four cases where his patients had been cured in a few days. Encouraged by this, Hall tried it on his own patients, who complained to him of severe pain for nine to twelve hours after each treatment, bleeding from the urethra, and great difficulty in urinating, none of which symptoms had been reported by Behrend. It is tempting to believe that Behrend's patients were declaring themselves cured in order to avoid further injections.

The painful effect of chloroform on sensitive membranes did not deter a doctor in a Spanish military hospital from treating a soldier's chronic inflammation of the eyelid with chloroform dropped directly into the eye. The doctor reported with some regret that he had been unable to effect a complete cure as the soldier could not be persuaded to remain in the hospital.[4]

Chloroform is an excellent solvent, a quality that ensures its place in the modern laboratory. In 1848, a preparation of the plant resin gutta-percha dissolved in chloroform was being used as a dressing to protect wounds and skin eruptions.[5] It was later marketed in Vienna under the name of Traumaticine.[6]

Despite its potential to cause irritation of the stomach, chloroform in dilute form was taken internally for a growing list of complaints. Its sedative action meant that it was extremely effective as an antidote for seasickness. Ingeniously, a Dr Edwin Chesshire suggested that the best preventative for sickness during operations under chloroform was chloroform itself, giving patients a few drops in water before commencing inhalation.[7]

Chloroform is only poorly soluble in water, and there were a variety of suggestions for suitable diluents, including liniment of soap, ether and glycerine. Simpson's recommendation was to mix it with oil, cream or soda water to abate nausea and vomiting and stop hiccups. In 1855 a M. Dannecy of Bordeaux suggested a rather pleasanter vehicle of almond oil, gum Arabic, syrup of orange flowers and water.[8]

A preparation that first became widely available in 1855 was Dr Collis Browne's chlorodyne – a name derived from chloroform anodyne. Its composition was a closely guarded secret, and there was a great deal of correspondence in the medical journals from doctors and chemists, each with his own recipe. While some doctors prescribed it, others resented both the extravagant claims for the product, which was said to relieve a wide variety of diseases, and the secrecy over its ingredients. The pleasant taste meant that patients, who were usually given a diluted mixture, were tempted to overdose, occasionally with fatal result. Its commercial success gave rise to some imitators, notably a Mr Freeman, who incautiously claimed to be the original inventor and was promptly sued. Unlike so many patent remedies of the time, chlorodyne continued its popularity with both doctors and patients for well over 100 years.

In 1862 it was suggested that the sweet taste of chloroform could be used to mask the bitterness of some medicines.[9] After some initial caution it was established that this would not reduce the effectiveness of the medication, and chloroform was adopted as a sweetener in many preparations. This use as a flavouring was to continue well into the twentieth century, in medicines, foodstuffs and confectionery.

In 1907 it was discovered that linseed liquorice and chlorodyne lozenges, which were widely consumed by both adults and children, contained dangerous amounts of chloroform. Ladies unwilling to enter a public house would consume them to achieve a pleasurable stupor, and schoolchilden who seemed dull and apathetic at their lessons improved markedly when their favourite sweets were taken away.[10]

In 1851 chloroform was hailed as a preservative of meat, when a M. Augend of Constantinople observed after a series of experiments that the dilute vapour would delay putrefaction.[11] It is not known if anyone actually sampled the meat so preserved, but over time, numerous experiments confirmed chloroform's excellent properties as a preservative of organic material.

CHLOROFORM AS A SEDATIVE

Spasmodic and convulsive conditions from persistent hiccups to cholera responded well to chloroform. Although it was not, as many claimed, a 'cure' it gave great relief from distressing symptoms, especially for those patients too ill to swallow opiates.

Soon after its introduction as an anaesthetic, medical journals began to record numerous testimonials from doctors on the efficiency with which chloroform produced relief in delirium tremens (seizures experienced by alcoholics following alcohol withdrawal), tetanus, strychnine poisoning, spasmodic asthma, bronchial cough, and rabies. The only effective treatment for rabies at the time was early cauterising of the animal bite with red-hot irons, which the patient dreaded as much as the disease. Chloroform meant that victims were more easily persuaded to take the treatment, and if convulsions did start, afforded much needed rest. In tetanus, chloroform saved lives by relaxing the muscular spasms of the throat that impeded breathing, and with frequent applications a fortunate patient might recover.

Where necessary, the administration of chloroform might be kept up for many hours or even days. In May 1853, a six-week-old child, suffering violent convulsions, was losing weight and obviously dying. As a last resort, chloroform was applied on a handkerchief, and reapplied whenever the effects wore off.

Occasionally the child was allowed to recover slightly, so it could feed. This continued for five days, and 16 ounces of chloroform were used. At the end of that time, the child was recovering and the fits did not return.[12]

Frequent dosing with chloroform did have one unlooked-for side-effect. In 1848 an eighteen-year-old girl in a Bristol hospital was thought to be dying from typhus (a painful infection transmitted by rat-borne fleas). Delirious, and worn out from lack of sleep, she was given chloroform, and after a peaceful rest, showed such improvement that the dose was repeated a number of times. By the time she was on her way to recovery, the girl had developed a craving for the treatment.[13] This was not an unusual reaction. Many patients were impressed not only by the efficacy of chloroform but its intoxicating delights. One lady, inhaling it for asthma, waved her arms about, and laughed hysterically, her prevailing impression being that she was riding on a moonbeam. She afterwards confessed that she had found the experience 'exceedingly pleasurable'.[14] If, after treatment ended, patients wished to obtain their own supply for a little private indulgence, a chemist would usually oblige.

One of the greatest scourges of the nineteenth century was cholera, the main symptoms of which were painful intestinal spasms, vomiting, and profuse watery diarrhoea. The specific for cholera in the 1840s was opium, but in a violent attack this could be vomited up before it could take effect, and patients would die of exhaustion and debility. Chloroform gave soothing relief from the terrible cramps, enabling the patient to take medication and nourishment. Even if a case was too far gone, it made the dying moments more peaceful.

Chloroform was also used to produce calm in other circumstances. In December 1847 a Mr Garner of St Ives was returning home with his horse and gig. During a brief stop to adjust the harness, the horse suddenly began to kick dangerously. Garner tried to hold the animal's head and bystanders rushed up to help, but the horse threw itself violently to the ground, with the exhausted man still holding on. At that moment, the local chemist, who had seen what was happening, rushed out with some chloroform on a handkerchief, and applied it to the horse's nostrils. Soon, the animal was insensible. The harness and gig were removed, and five minutes later the horse got up, shook itself and was led quietly into the stable.[15]

What chloroform could do for an animal it could also do in man, and it soon became a valuable standby of asylums, to be used on the violent insane. It was not always possible to have a doctor in attendance when it was needed, so it was often applied by people with no medical qualifications. In 1860 a female lunatic died after chloroform was given to her by the workhouse governor to control fits of mania.[16] In America in 1866 a prisoner under sentence of death was in a state of such wild excitement that no one dared enter his cell and the sheriff called in the aid of a medical man who syringed chloroform on to the prisoner through the grating of the door until he was sufficiently sedated for the irons to be put on him.[17] In New York in 1869 a convicted murderer was hanged while under the influence of chloroform. It was applied as he stood on the drop, which, with nice timing, fell as soon as he became insensible.[18]

Patients were often very talkative under chloroform, and in 1864, Dr Sédillot of Strasbourg tested its ability as a truth drug by asking patients to try not to reply to questions as they were coming out of anaesthesia. They invariably failed, and the law duly took note.[19] In 1870 the *Lancet* reported that a man in New York had murdered his wife, a neighbour and the neighbour's son. On being arrested, he feigned insanity. He was chloroformed, much against his will, and when questioned immediately on awakening, answered questions truthfully. When he realised what he had done, a full confession followed.[20]

Chloroform was also used by army surgeons to detect feigned diseases such as pretended paralysis, contraction of the limbs and deafness. Initially some army surgeons believed that chloroform would induce an epileptic fit, and could be used to detect a fraud,[21] but Snow, who found the idea distasteful, said he had given it to epileptics with no ill effects.[22]

LOCAL ANAESTHESIA

Although it was recognised soon after its introduction that chloroform caused blistering when left in contact with the skin, there were numerous attempts to use it as a local anaesthetic. In 1848 Professor Simpson was busy carrying out a series of experiments on animals.[23] In one procedure he placed a few drops of chloroform in a tumbler, pasted paper over its mouth, and made a hole in the cover into which he inserted the rear half of a centipede. Once the chloroform had taken effect he removed the centipede, which crawled about on its front legs, dragging its last few segments behind it, from which the legs dangled motionless. As Simpson watched, it recovered its powers of movement segment by segment.

Moving on to mammals, Simpson placed the back leg of a rabbit into a bladder containing chloroform vapour and left it there for an hour. He then tried pinching and squeezing both back legs to compare reactions. This showed some anaesthetic effect, but when he tried galvanism, the animal cried with pain. He repeated this experiment with a guinea-pig, placing the whole of its hind quarters in the bladder, and comparing pain reactions on the front and back. Unfortunately the chloroform caused severe redness and congestion to the tissues.

His human experiments, mainly on himself, included rubbing chloroform on the gums, which he thought was effective and of potential use to dentists. Wrapping his hand in a handkerchief soaked with chloroform was less successful, and caused reddening and burning of the skin. He doubted that many people would be able to keep their hand in contact with liquid chloroform for long, although on one occasion he kept his hand in a jar of chloroform for an hour, and one of his pupils, a Mr Adams, had managed two hours. Placing his hand in a jar of chloroform vapour also produced local anaesthesia, but reddened his skin, and the effect was never enough to allow an operation requiring a deep incision.

Simpson also applied chloroform to the inside of his lips, his tongue and even his eyes, but found that with mucous surfaces the heat and burning were too intense to allow long contact. He knew that Nunneley had reported performing an eye operation after applying chloroform vapour for 20 minutes, and the eye had been swollen and painful for some time afterwards.[24] Simpson and Duncan tried this but also found that their eyes became red and painful and they could not tolerate the undiluted vapour for longer than two or three minutes.

In France there was considerable interest in chloroform as a local application for minor complaints. It was also used to relieve post-operative pain, by applying it directly to the cut surface after amputation.[25] Orchitis (painful swelling of the testicles) was treated with a compress of cloth dipped in chloroform, applied to the scrotum in a suspensory bandage, and renewed every three hours,[26] while a Dr Dumont reported that he had subdued a case of satyriasis in a no doubt grateful 46-year-old priest by topical applications of chloroform.[27] In Paris in 1854 some experiments were made blowing chloroform vapour on to the skin before operations to remove abscesses, but this did not meet with much success.[28]

Dentists soon discovered that the pain of a rotten tooth could be soothed by packing the cavity with cotton wool soaked in chloroform, and also recommended rubbing it on the gums. On one occasion, Professor Simpson was on an excursion with his youngest son and called in at a chemist's shop to buy some chloroform to treat the boy's toothache. The cautious chemist refused to sell him any, saying that he did not sell it to folk who knew nothing about it.[29]

Chloroform vapour was also applied by douche for painful conditions of the vagina. In 1854, Dr Hardy of Dublin patented a special apparatus for this purpose,[30] but Simpson treated period pains using an ordinary enema syringe, which he thought superior. In some cases, he declared that chloroform had done more than give temporary relief; it had actually cured the condition. He had also seen the vapour injected into the rectum for irritability and painful spasms.[31]

Chloroform was incorporated into many lotions and ointments for general application in painful conditions. In France, a simple preparation of 60 drops of chloroform to an ounce of hog's lard was used. For rigidity of the cervix in labour Simpson advised an ointment of chloroform in lard or butter. In 1857 a Professor Rusponi discovered that shaking up chloroform with raw egg-white produced a gelatinous mixture which could be spread on linen and used as a poultice.[32]

For a time it seemed that there was no sphere of life that chloroform could not transform. In 1849 tests carried out in France suggested that both chloroform and ether were very effective in supplying the motive power for steamships.[33] Four years later it was reported that the inhabitants of the port of Lorient had just witnessed a test run by the chloroform-powered 120-hp steamer *Galilee* under the inspection of the Minister of Marine. The steamer made several turns around the harbour, achieving a rate of 9 knots and it was declared that the success of the experiment was complete.[34] History records nothing more, so it seems that despite the promising start, chloroform power never really took off.

VETERINARY PRACTICE

The application of anaesthetics to valued animals brought its own special problems. One difficulty of chloroforming a horse was the potential for injury as it fell. Pearson Ferguson, a vet, solved the problem by first having the horse cast (placed in a position where it could not get its legs under it). He placed a piece of chloroform-soaked sponge in its left nostril, then produced the effects of an inhaler by the simple expedient of covering the horse's right nostril with his hand as it inhaled, and then covering the left when it exhaled.[35] Other vets tried a different approach, first hobbling the horse, and creating a nosebag-like inhaler with a soaked sponge inside. As the horse lost consciousness, the hobbles were drawn up enabling a fall that would not injure the animal.[36]

In 1850 a leopard which had been presented to the London Zoo by the Pasha of Egypt suffered an accident in its cage which resulted in a compound fracture of the leg. Professor Simmonds of the Royal Veterinary College was consulted and decided that amputation was necessary to save the animal's life. The question then arose of how to chloroform a leopard, the answer being, very carefully, with a sponge on the end of a long stick. After some protests it succumbed, and eventually made a full recovery.[37]

In 1855 a 120-year-old elephant at Mr Wombwell's menagerie was unable to walk due to diseased feet, and it was decided that it should be humanely destroyed. A veterinary surgeon and a chemist were sent for, and administered chloroform. How much they used was not recorded, but in ten minutes the animal became insensible. They then injected prussic acid and strychnine, but after a while it was clear that this was having no effect. It was decided to continue with the chloroform in the hope that the animal might die from this alone, but after three hours it seemed to have made no difference at all. The administration was stopped, and an hour and half later the animal had fully recovered. After further consultation, it was decided that the old methods were the best, but the elephant was again chloroformed, before a bullet divided an artery, which was further opened with a knife. This was perhaps not as clean a death as originally planned, but in a few minutes the animal expired without struggle or pain.[38]

THE FIRST TWO DECADES OF CHLOROFORM

The introduction of anaesthesia led, as was hoped, to a steady increase in the amount and complexity of surgery, and a decrease in amputations, as lengthier and more conservative procedures were possible. Most of Europe and much of the United States preferred chloroform to ether, but despite the best efforts of the medical profession deaths from chloroform anaesthesia continued with depressing regularity. Medical journals were inundated with letters on the correct method of administration of chloroform, from doctors who were convinced that deaths were avoidable if only everyone followed their advice. Unfortunately, there was considerable disagreement as to how anaesthetics affected the patient, a plethora of opinions on what caused deaths, and any number of methods of resuscitation. What some recommended was denounced as useless or even dangerous by others, and the result was a confusing mass of conflicting information.

One opponent of chloroform, Dr James Arnott, mangled the death statistics to promote his method of 'congelation', or local anaesthesia, by freezing mixtures of ice and salt. Arnott insisted that surgical deaths were greater since chloroform had been introduced, but he attributed all deaths to chloroform, and ignored the increase in surgery.[39] He was convinced that chloroform would soon be abandoned, and replaced with his system, but in the event it was congelation which fell by the wayside, to be superseded by the ether spray.

Arnott's belief that deaths from chloroform were more numerous than supposed may not have been far from the truth. In April 1854, the *Lancet* commented drily that a French journal had reported the first chloroform death in France, and suggested that this was only the first because the earlier ones had been put down to other causes.[40] Arnott had also made the valid point that cases where a patient had stopped breathing and been revived were not included in the statistics of chloroform accidents. While doctors mentioned these occurrences, usually to congratulate themselves on their skill at resuscitation, no official record was maintained. 'Deaths from chloroform are now becoming a kind of unfortunate casualty which, like shipwrecks and railway accidents, may from time to time be expected,' said the *Lancet*, citing fatty degeneration of the heart as a cause of death, and wondering how it could be detected in a living person.[41] The editor believed that the use of chloroform should be restricted. Referring to a recent death he asked, 'Was the intensity or duration of the pain in an amputation of the leg sufficient to justify the fatal risk in such a subject? Or can it be said that insensibility was essential to the surgeon's proceedings? Surely not.'[42]

The *Lancet* was particularly outraged at the use of chloroform in dentistry. When a young woman died in the dentist's chair at Epsom in 1858, the editor uttered a stern warning, in terms it believed no one could ignore. 'It is chiefly our fashionable ladies who demand chloroform. This time it was a servant girl who was sacrificed; the next time it may be a Duchess.'[43]

The *Lancet* could not fail to notice that most reported deaths occurred when chloroform was administered on a handkerchief. There were no statistics on the relative popularity of different methods of administration, but the *Lancet* decided that the handkerchief method was inherently dangerous, and urged repeatedly over the course of several years that the best guarantee of safety was using an inhaler. Snow's device and its later modifications were particularly recommended.

Lectures given by Simpson in 1854 show that he was by then admitting that chloroform deaths did occur, but believed that these were extremely rare, and not necessarily attributable to 'that pain-annulling agent'. In Edinburgh, he claimed (probably on the basis of the amount of chloroform manufactured) that there had only been one death in 500,000 administrations, a wonderful record if it had been true.[44] He distinguished two modes of death – asphyxia, from the cloth being applied for too long, and sudden syncope, mentioning the case of a woman who prior to the operation had been subject to fainting fits. The first kind was clearly the fault of the doctor and the second was due to idiosyncrasy and therefore the fault of the patient.

Dr Protheroe Smith, an ardent admirer of Simpson, thought he had found a safer way of administering chloroform.[45] Retiring one night into his dressing room with a syringe full of chloroform vapour, he removed his lower garments and injected the contents of the syringe into his rectum. Anaesthesia was rapid and profound, so much so that when he awoke lying on the floor, half naked and shivering, he had no recollection of how he had got there. Groping around behind him, his hand encountered the syringe, and memory came flooding back. The inflammation and copious diarrhoea that followed ensured that he did not repeat the experiment, and Simpson took the experience as sufficient discouragement not to try it, although he obviously relished relating the story in his lectures.

After ten years of anaesthesia, with the profession no further forward in the fraught matter of avoiding chloroform deaths, the early euphoria had vanished. In July 1858 Professor Miller addressed the Annual General Meeting of the British Medical Association, in a very different vein from his original eulogistic paper of 1848. While still believing that chloroform was safe for children he added:

> In the case of adults . . . compete anaesthesia by inhalation ought to be had recourse to only in obedience to the requirement of stern necessity . . . in any minor procedure . . . I would be slow to humour the patient's fancy. When chloroform was first brought into use I was a great enthusiast in its praise. I esteemed it to be as safe and manageable as it was beneficial, and thought that it could hardly be used too often or too freely . . . subsequent events have chastened and subdued my tone.[46]

The shock of witnessing the sudden death of a patient was enough to make a doctor radically change his notions, as did Bristol surgeon Augustin Pritchard who stated, 'I venture to prophesy that anaesthesia will more and more fall into disuse, and ultimately be had recourse to only for the most severe or protracted operations.'[47]

Ten years later, it was still felt that anaesthesia was contra-indicated for certain procedures. There was considerable prejudice against the use of chloroform in eye operations, as it was feared that violent vomiting would eject the fluid part of the eye. Experience would show that not only were these fears unjustified, but the profound relaxation produced by chloroform was especially beneficial. In 1868 Thomas Radford was performing caesarean operations without chloroform, which he felt would affect the contractions of the uterus, and praised the fortitude of his patients.[48] That year saw the visit to London of Dr Colton, who had revived the use of nitrous oxide. Although the duration of the anaesthesia it produced made it unsuitable for prolonged operations, London dentists rapidly adopted it, with a consequent fall in the death rate.

After the death of John Snow, another quiet man who liked to make careful measurements, Joseph Clover, became the leading anaesthetist in England. Born in 1825, he ultimately became a lecturer in anaesthetics at University College Hospital, and chloroformist to the Westminster Hospital and the London Dental Hospital. Originally destined for a medical career, poor health due to chronic lung disease had diverted him to the less arduous role of specialist anaesthetist, in which he excelled. Clover's great talent was his ability to translate the desire for the meticulous administration of measured doses of chloroform into a practical apparatus. He devised an inhaler in 1862 which was a considerable improvement on Snow's 'bag and bellows', overcoming the problem of the large air-bag getting in the way by wearing it slung over his shoulder. He used concertina bellows containing exactly 1,000 cubic inches of air to charge the bag, and to each bellowsful he added by glass syringe 32 minims of chloroform, which produced 37 cubic inches of vapour. By 1868 he had administered it in 1,700 cases without fatal result. In operations on the teeth and jaws he would first induce anaesthesia with a face-piece, then remove it and replace it with a cap that fitted closely over the nose, judicious pressure on the bag ensuring that the mixture was inhaled. Clover's apparatus soon became the *Lancet*'s inhaler of choice, and the experimental work of the Royal Medical and Chirurgical Society was carried out under his guidance. His confidence and expertise dispelled anxiety, and his sympathetic manner and lack of ostentation earned him many friends. Unlike John Snow, however, Clover was never to assemble a list of cases or leave to the profession a work collecting all his considerable experience, but during his lifetime he was a highly influential figure in his field.

Established medical opinions were slow to change, and deaths continued to be reported as due to fatty degeneration of the heart, even in patients in their teens or twenties. Doctors expected to see it, and often searched for it microscopically, sometimes observing small fatty deposits in the tissues, which they assumed were a pre-existing condition and responsible for the death.

In 1860 Simpson changed the way he administered chloroform. It was a simple modification, but it became very popular, and gave rise to a completely new breed of mask. For thirteen years Simpson had used a folded cloth soaked in chloroform which was held over the patient's nose and mouth, keeping his hand between the cloth and the face of the patient in order to admit sufficient air. He now used a single layer of fabric, which was laid dry in a concave shape over the patient's nose and mouth. The chloroform was then applied to the fabric drop by drop. He found that there was very little waste, as the chloroform was inhaled as soon as it touched the fabric. The thin layer easily admitted sufficient air. This came to be known as the 'open drop method'. Simpson was unable to resist a comment on the essential safety of chloroform:

> I have often feared lest the lives of patients should be sacrificed by the careless manner in which, in particular, students and young practitioners sometimes employ the damp folded cloth over the patient's face without admitting a sufficient supply of air; and no doubt many of the deaths attributed to chloroform are due only to the improper administration of it, and are consequently no more chargeable on the drug itself than are the many deaths resulting from overdoses of opium, etc.[49]

The only precaution Simpson advised was that, since the face of the patient would be in close contact with the wet fabric, the lips and nose should first be anointed with oil or ointment.

In May 1862, Dr Thomas Skinner, who had worked with Simpson, introduced a new concept to the obstetrical society of London.[50] It was simple, cheap, and portable, and seemed to combine the best features of both inhaler and handkerchief. His mask was a simple oval wire frame, with a handle for the operator to hold, and its domed shape meant that when it was covered with fabric, nothing could touch the face of the patient, and air was freely admitted. It was used with a single layer of material, and the chloroform was applied with a dropper bottle. Two versions were manufactured, one which was carried in a leather case, and one designed to be folded away in the doctor's hat. The Skinner mask, as it came to be known, was the precursor of many variations on the basic design, which changed little over the next forty years.

By 1863 it had become apparent that despite every variation on administration, and pre-operative checks of the patient's condition, deaths were still occurring with alarming frequency. Early confidence that children were in some way immune had been shattered by a number of deaths, just as sudden, and for similar minor procedures as in adults. The medical profession clamoured for official guidance, and in 1863 the Royal Medical and Chirurgical Society set up a committee to study the use of chloroform in three situations: the treatment of disease, in surgery, and in midwifery.[51] Doctors were asked to supply the following information:

1. Reports of unpublished cases of death from chloroform or any other anaesthetic
2. More complete reports of fatal cases already reported
3. Notes of accidents in which death was threatened but averted
4. The effects when employed by inhalation for the remedial treatment of disease
5. Comparative results of operations both before and after the introduction of anaesthesia

The report was not published until July 1864.[52] Seventy meetings had been held and numerous experiments carried out. The result was, to say the least, inconclusive. The committee found that chloroform deaths were due to failure of both the heart and respiration, and recommended that no more than a 3.5 per cent concentration of vapour be used. Ether was thought to be safer than chloroform, but slower and less certain in producing anaesthesia. The committee did not therefore advise a return to ether but suggested a mixture of alcohol, chloroform and ether. No specific apparatus was recommended, indeed, contrary to the *Lancet*'s official view, doctors were told that an apparatus was not necessary if care was taken. How one was supposed to ensure that the dilution was no more than 3.5 per cent when using a handkerchief was not indicated. The committee also found that there had been no instances of death from chloroform in the United Kingdom during natural labour. However, the eagerly awaited report was an obvious disappointment. It did not give the clarity doctors had hoped for, and such suggestions as it did make were immediately challenged.

Dr Charles Kidd, a medical reporter who witnessed many thousands of operations, had no faith in mixtures. The 1863 committee had assumed that when chloroform, ether and alcohol were mixed, their vapours arose in the same proportion as the mixture, but Kidd said that this was not the case.[53] Extensive trials abroad had shown that the ether was inhaled first then the chloroform, leaving the alcohol behind. He recommended the use of ether and chloroform, not mixed, but given alternately. Kidd also pointed out that in animal experiments death was always by deliberate overdose. He didn't doubt that large doses killed animals, but human deaths appeared to take place under light anaesthesia. This apparent paradox was ignored by many and espoused by few, but it formed a common thread of debate in chloroform history, and was not resolved for many years.

In 1866 a Dr Robert Ellis tried to overcome the mixture problem with an apparatus which vaporised the fluids in separate chambers and then combined the vapour in regulated proportions, a system which anticipated the modern anaesthetic array. Ellis, clearly bursting with pride under a becoming mask of modesty, introduced his apparatus to the profession, but to his surprise it was coolly dismissed. Doctors who liked the simplicity of the handkerchief, or had their own inhalers to promote, did not want to be 'encumbered with too many mechanical complications'.[54]

For some years hospitals had informally employed doctors who specialised in anaesthesia, but in 1864 the *Lancet* was able to applaud the formal recognition of this duty by the decision to appoint specialist chloroformists. In 1865, the Westminster Hospital announced that Mr Clover would administer chloroform to all surgical patients. He would also give instruction to the resident officers, so they would be capable of acting in his absence, and give lectures on the administration of chloroform.

While Clover demonstrated his bag and bellows in London, another figure was emerging from the Scottish scene who would later achieve international fame, and exercise a considerable influence over the chloroform debate. Joseph Lister had visited Edinburgh in 1853 and struck up what was to become a lifelong friendship with James Syme. Staying on, he became Syme's house-surgeon, ardent supporter and in 1856 his son-in-law. By 1860 he was Professor of Surgery at Glasgow, and it was here he began the work which was to lead to his development of the antiseptic system of surgery, which was violently opposed by Simpson. In 1869, the man who had been so enraged at others' blind refusal to accept chloroform denounced Lister's use of carbolic acid: 'Was there ever a higher delusion than seeing men – rational men, anointing their knives and saws with it?'[55]

Many honours came to Simpson, the greatest of which was a baronetcy in 1866, but he never ceased his search for new anaesthetics. Sir Lyon (later Baron) Playfair (professor of chemistry at the University of Edinburgh from 1858 to 1868) once recalled how Simpson had come to his laboratory wanting to test a potential anaesthetic. Playfair had resisted Simpson's demands that he test it on himself and tried it instead on two rabbits, one of which died.[56]

Despite the publicity given to chloroform deaths in both national and local press it continued to be popular with patients who had come to expect anaesthesia for surgery as a matter of right. In 1869, William Godley, a 25-year-old Sheffield chemist, required an operation for removal of a diseased leg bone. Having read the medical journals he was well acquainted with the risks and declared that he was sure it would go badly with him. Nevertheless he was determined to have an anaesthetic, so, in a highly anxious state, fortified with beef tea and wine, he submitted to the chloroform. Three minutes later he suddenly sat up, threw out his arms, and fell back, dead.[57]

Those members of the public without the benefit of Godley's knowledge appeared to believe that a healthy constitution would insure them against danger, or that if they had taken chloroform once without ill effect they could do so safely again. In 1864 William Lavis, a 26-year-old Devon carpenter with an injured foot, chose to have an operation to remove dead bone rather than wait for it to detach naturally. 'Don't give me too much,' he said, as 40 minims of chloroform were poured into the inhaler. They were his last words.[58]

Herbert Hildyard Clarke of Lincoln College Oxford, who required a minor operation, was first asked if he was able to take chloroform. 'Of course I can!' he exclaimed, having taken it once before. He was seated in a chair, and a few drops were applied on some wool in a handkerchief. He leaped to his feet in wild agitation, and it was necessary to restrain him, then he fell to the ground. He was lifted into the chair, and the operation was performed, but the pallor that spread over his face announced his death. The post-mortem suggested that despite an outward appearance of health he had an enlarged heart. He was nineteen.[59]

Edinburgh's reputation for safety was from time to time shown up for the myth it was. In 1865 a lady of that city asked her dentist to give her chloroform for a tooth extraction. She had had it before without harm, and it was Edinburgh, after all. He declined on the grounds that he had had a fatality in his practice quite recently. This was insufficient warning and she went to her own doctor insisting he give her chloroform, and he agreed. She was young, she was healthy, and, very soon, she was dead.[60]

Despite these and many similar reports from all over the world, Sir James Young Simpson remained a believer in chloroform to the last, and inhaled it for relief from the chronic angina which began to affect him in 1868. Worn out with years of overwork and self-experimentation, his heart gave up the struggle in May 1870. His death provoked national mourning – the flags of the country flew at half-mast for the funeral, and Queen Victoria sent a personal message of sympathy to the family. The house in Queen Street is now a centre for drugs counselling and related services, and the ground floor dining-room where the properties of chloroform were so dramatically discovered has been preserved in its original style.

Syme died only two months later in July 1870, but in the previous year, his prestigious Edinburgh chair of surgery had passed to Joseph Lister, who became the new champion of the Scottish method of giving chloroform.

Elsewhere, however, confidence in chloroform was on the decline. Doctors who had once been certain that medical science would soon guarantee the safe use of chloroform were still unable either to predict or prevent distressing deaths of mainly youthful and vigorous patients. Not only was there nothing better to put in its place, there seemed no likelihood that there ever would be.

SEVEN

Chloroform Goes to War

> In desperate wounds of the extremities . . . will any thinking man again give chloroform? . . . We think – we hope not. Common sense will surely teach us better, and notwithstanding the many plausible reasons in favour of chloroform, prevent us from committing an error which has hastened many a fellow-being to the grave.
>
> *John Jones Cole, surgeon, Punjab war, 1852*[1]

In March 1855, a Dr William Philpot Brookes observed that recent consignments of medical supplies sent to the Crimea omitted one essential item – chloroform. This he put down not to shortages or even incompetence – he believed it was a deliberate act by the military medical authorities to prevent surgeons using chloroform when operating on the wounded. He may well have been right.[2]

On the face of it, chloroform, apart from its tendency to cause occasional sudden death in minor surgery, is admirably suited for the battlefield. In 1855, the only real alternative was ether, which was highly inflammable. Ether was also slower to take effect, a matter of vital importance in front-line hospitals where casualties could be pouring in faster than it was possible to deal with them. Ether had a greater tendency to make patients thrash around uncontrollably during administration, which was hazardous where there were severe injuries such as compound fractures. The relatively small volume of chloroform required to anaesthetise a patient was a boon when facilities for carrying and storing supplies were limited. It is not surprising that the reintroduction of nitrous oxide, which required special equipment and storage, did nothing to challenge the supremacy of chloroform on the battlefield. Despite the obvious advantages, however, it took time for chloroform to be generally accepted for use by military surgeons, for there was concern amounting sometimes to dogmatic insistence that anaesthetics were harmful to patients with gunshot or shellfire wounds, who would be in a state of shock. Chloroform was known to depress the action of the heart, and badly injured men therefore needed a stimulant, one of the most readily available stimulants being pain. Since causes of death were often difficult to determine, both the advocates and opponents of chloroform could cite cases that supported their views, and there was the inevitable theorising on what would have happened in any given case under different treatment. It was true that military surgeons had a far greater experience of major injuries than those in civilian life, a fact that they often mentioned as evidence of their authority, yet the average surgeon did sometimes deal with wounds from firearms, or from serious accidents, and saw no reason to believe that military injuries were any different.

The conditions under which military surgery was carried out in the mid-nineteenth century were unpleasant and dangerous to both patient and surgeon. A field hospital might have been no more than a tent, situated hopefully but not invariably out of range of shell and shot. Surgery was often performed in the open air on whatever flat surface was available or could be improvised, within sight and sound of those who had just been operated upon and those who were waiting their turn. Sometimes a building was commandeered for hospital use, and this could be a far less sanitary option, coming as it often did with a resident infestation. The operating table might be a door, torn off its hinges and laid across packing cases, or failing that, the ground. Hygiene was virtually non-existent, and the instrument of choice for probing gunshot wounds was the surgeon's finger. The almost inevitable infections were considered to be normal, and doctors spoke approvingly of wounds 'suppurating healthily'.

CHLOROFORM MARCHES OUT

The first use of anaesthesia in battlefield surgery was during the United States–Mexico war. Texas had declared itself independent from Mexico in 1835, and when the United States admitted Texas into the Union in 1845, conflict soon followed. War was officially declared on 13 May 1846 and the final peace was signed on 4 July

1848, thus spanning the period from before inhalation anaesthesia through the introduction of ether and the arrival of chloroform.

In March 1847 Dr E.H. Barton visited the hospital at Vera Cruz, bringing both ether and the apparatus to administer it, and made a successful demonstration,[3] but the Surgeon-General, Dr Thomas Lawson, thought it too volatile, and the equipment too fragile for military use.[4] In charge of the hospital was Surgeon John B. Porter, who had no time for the new invention. In a war where the death rate from disease was ten times higher than that from enemy action, Porter blamed anaesthesia for blood poisoning, haemorrhage, muscle damage, and gangrene. He even claimed that hospital gangrene had not existed before anaesthesia.[5] Lawson was flexible enough to see the advantages of anaesthesia, even if he was unconvinced about ether, and after the introduction of chloroform he ordered it for army use.

Porter's beliefs had a far-reaching effect on both American and European opinion. Dr Arnott, as part of his campaign for the acceptance of congelation, later quoted the 'conviction of Dr Porter of the American army that in the cases in which he saw anaesthetics employed during the late war with Mexico they exercised a decidedly unfavourable influence upon the state of the wounds and upon the result of the operation'.[6] It was this kind of comment in the widely read medical press that gave many doctors doubts about chloroform when their turn came to use it on the battlefield.

Chloroform was already widely used in France, when in February 1848, economic depression in France led to street fighting in Paris. Dr Velpeau, who less than ten years previously had been resigned to the permanent inseparability of pain and surgery, treated numerous gunshot wounds, but caution led him to advise that anaesthetics should not be used in such cases.[7] Four months later, however, experience had changed his mind. In June 1848, violent protests in Paris lasted three days and were repressed by the military. Over a thousand people were killed, and many thousands more were wounded. Dr Charles Kidd was there, sent by the *Medical Times* to report on the surgery, and saw some 1,600 operations carried out under chloroform by the eminent surgeons of the day, including Velpeau.[8]

Many British surgeons served in India and used chloroform on both European and native casualties, the first major conflict in which it was used being the second Sikh war in 1848–9. The

British East India Company had expanded its control over the sub-continent in the early nineteenth century, occupying the Punjab in 1846. A revolt against the British led to several bloody and ultimately decisive battles in early 1849 when the Sikh forces were finally defeated. John Jones Cole, surgeon to the auxiliary forces in the Punjab had very decisive views on chloroform. Born in 1817, Cole had qualified as a surgeon before the introduction of anaesthesia, and was a firm believer that pain was 'one of the most powerful, one of the most salutary *stimulants known*', and that chloroform was 'injurious in field practice'.[9] He describes the following incident in his textbook on military surgery:

> I had established a large hospital in the city of Mooltan, for the reception of the enemy's wounded. One morning, in going round, I noticed a man whose stump was being dressed, and was informed that a friend, who was in the habit of coming to my assistance, had amputated his thigh the evening before. I pointed out how well the operation had been performed, but added, feeling the patient's pulse, that he would not recover. Soon after, I met my friend, and said, 'I have seen your handiwork, up there, and a better or cleaner stump I have not often noticed. You will not, however, save your man.' 'Indeed! Why, he is a fine, strong fellow.' 'Ah, but he looks as if he had taken *chloroform*.' 'Chloroform! We gave it him before the operation, and he did not suffer the slightest pain.' 'Did you? Then your patient's hours are numbered.' He died before the evening.[10]

Cole's advice to doctors – to put the chloroform bottle away on a high shelf, and if the weather was hot, leave the stopper out to keep it cool – must surely have been mischievous! Whether he would have changed his opinions with time is not known, for he died in India in 1855.

Others, however, were more enthusiastic. William Barker M'Egan, assistant surgeon to His Highness the Nizam's 2nd regiment of cavalry Mominabad, wrote to the *Lancet* in 1851 to describe the effects of chloroform on native casualties. M'Egan had used chloroform on numerous casualties without ill effect. He had originally been of the opinion that Indians were more likely to be unfavourably affected by chloroform than Europeans, yet found this not to be the case. In his letter he described a skirmish in which 'I accompanied my regiment into action having my horse cut down from under me, so that we doctors are not at all times exempt from the good things going.'

There were forty-nine enemy wounded and he performed eighteen amputations. Only three men died, at a time when he might have expected 50 per cent fatalities, and when he wrote the letter some of the patients had recovered enough to fight against the British again.[11] M'Egan, who was born in 1817, later served at Scutari and with the Turkish contingent in the Crimea, before returning to India. He and his wife had the misfortune to be in Jhansi in 1857 when the mutineers murdered the white residents.[12]

NEW CHALLENGES

In September 1854, French and British troops were sent to the Crimean peninsula. Earlier that year, Russian forces had been driven from the occupied Turkish territories, and it was decided to press home the advantage by destroying the Russian naval base at Sebastopol. For British forces it was the first major European conflict since 1815, and there was a new threat to contend with, the conical bullet, which produced far more damaging injuries than the round musket ball.

In 1854, the two standard texts on military medicine were written by men whose careers as army surgeons had ended nearly forty years previously, and both said remarkably little about chloroform. George James Guthrie referred to it only once, in his final paragraph:

> Chloroform, which has been recommended in all the great operations as a general rule, sometimes proves fatal, when incautiously administered or its use too long continued. In America chloric ether has been found equally efficient and less dangerous. It should therefore be brought into more general use and its qualities fully determined.[13]

The best one can say about this is that it recommends caution, but he surely meant to refer to 'sulphuric ether' in America, and the last sentence really doesn't make it clear which agent he is recommending.

Sir George Ballingall mentions chloroform twice, to commend its use in treating dislocations, and exposing cases of feigned contraction of the joints. The chapter on amputation, which is admittedly entirely technical in nature, makes no mention of anaesthesia at all.[14]

British medical opinion on the military use of chloroform was severely polarised. Young doctors, who had encountered it in medical schools and were confident in its use, saw every reason to employ it in the field, while to older surgeons, who regarded it with distrust, it was wholly unsuitable. The stage was set for a major row, and it erupted in September. Supplies of chloroform had been sent both to army and navy surgeons for the earlier campaign, but on 17 June 1854 the veteran Dr John Hall arrived in Turkey to take charge of hospital services. With the armies due to land in the Crimea, he had some important preparatory advice for Dr Andrew Smith, Director General of the Army Medical Department:

> Dr Hall takes this opportunity of cautioning medical officers against the use of chloroform in the severe shock of gunshot wounds, as he thinks few will survive where it is used. But as public opinion, founded perhaps on mistaken philanthropy, he knows is against him, he can only caution medical officers and entreat they will narrowly watch its effect; for however barbarous it may appear, the smart of the knife is a powerful stimulant: and it is much better to hear a man bawl lustily than to see him sink silently into the grave.[15]

This directive, issued on 3 September 1854 and published in the *Illustrated London News* on the 23rd, outraged most of the medical staff. Hall, fifty-nine at the time, had been a military medical officer since 1815. He was a man of very great experience in many parts of the world where he had served with diligence and distinction, and there is no doubt that he was stating what he believed was for the best. Nevertheless, he was severely out of touch. Early in the campaign, his failure to report shortages of supplies at Scutari misled the army medical department in England into thinking that all was well, and when Florence Nightingale arrived, he opposed her at every turn, and persistently tried to get her sent back home.

Graphic accounts of suffering caused by the woeful lack of supplies and personnel reached England in letters sent by army doctors and soldiers to family and friends back home, and they knew exactly what to do. They sent the letters to *The Times* and *The Times* published them. A few days later reprints appeared in other newspapers. Men inspired by tales of valour, who had sailed to the Crimea dreaming of glory and medals, had died racked with cholera before even seeing the enemy. Gallant soldiers, torn in battle, lay neglected for days with untended festering wounds, were jolted on bullock carts for want of proper transport, and lacked the most basic medicines and comforts. It was a shock to the nation and distressing to those whose menfolk were at the Crimea. 'We sit at home,' said a sad letter, 'trying to picture the last moments of those dear to us, and our agony is increased by the fear that all was not done that might have been done to relieve their sufferings, or, may be, to save their lives.'[16]

When on 12 October *The Times* published a leading article[17] suggesting that gentlemen reading their newspapers by the fireside might consider what they could do for their fellow countrymen, the response was immediate. Outraged at government blunders, citizens of every rank of society dug deep in their pockets, and the very next day the cheques, one of them from Sir Robert Peel in the sum of £200, poured in.

Hall's directive found little favour in Edinburgh, and Professor Syme responded in a letter to *The Times*:[18]

> Chloroform does not increase the danger of operations performed during a state of exhaustion, however extreme . . . pain instead of being a 'powerful stimulant', most injuriously exhausts the nervous energy of a weak patient . . . therefore, so far as the safety of operations may be in question, chloroform proves useful directly in proportion to the severity of the injury or disease and the degree of exhaustion or shock.

Dr Hall was not without his supporters, however. Someone signing himself 'A Military Surgeon' dashed off a reply to *The Times*, which was printed the following day:

> As Professor Syme's letter in *The Times* today, however well intended, may give pain to the relatives of our brave soldiers in the Crimea, by raising a suspicion of the judgement of the principal medical authority there on a very important point in military surgery, may I beg permission to state that Mr Syme's

> opinion . . . is in direct opposition to the general opinion of the profession, and the rules usually laid down for the administration of this substance?[19]

The letter goes on to advocate the use of numbing with cold, which leads to the strong suspicion that this was James Arnott putting his oar in.

Dr Richard Mackenzie, an able and enthusiastic young surgeon of Edinburgh, took the view that even if there was some risk with chloroform in the case of gunshot wounds, surgeons had the sense to use it wisely. He had studied under Simpson and Syme, and ensured that a bottle of chloroform was among the essential supplies he packed before leaving for the East, later reporting, 'Dr Hall's order is to discourage the use of it altogether. No one, I think should take any notice of it.'[20].

The first major battle of the campaign was at Alma in September, where Mackenzie treated the wounded with shellfire whizzing over his head, only to succumb to cholera a few days later. (His death left a vacant post in Edinburgh, which was filled by a rising young doctor called Joseph Lister.) The army then prepared to besiege Sebastopol, two more conflicts being fought at Inkerman and Balaclava. Chloroform was used for amputations, but supplies were scarce. Only 8 ounces were available for each regiment, and some surgeons were forced to borrow from others' meagre stocks.[21] Field surgeons sent favourable reports of the action of chloroform to the medical journals, which helped to turn the tide of opinion.

When surgeon E.M. Wrench arrived in November, morale was at its lowest ebb, for a supply ship carrying medicine and warm clothing had just been sunk in a hurricane. He observed that older surgeons had a great dread of chloroform, fostered by Hall's directive: 'We therefore only used chloroform for the more serious operations, and never to facilitate examination or for what we considered trivial operations, as cutting out bullets or setting fractures.'[22]

In March 1855 Andrew Smith supported Hall in giving evidence to a parliamentary committee that in cases of gunshot wounds requiring amputation 'the depressing effects of chloroform would render recovery of the man less probable than that of a man who underwent the operation without the chloroform.'[23]

Civilian practitioners such as Dr William Philpot Brookes

disagreed: 'I am sorry to see the heads of the army medical department continue their antiquated notions. . . .'[24]

In the wake of public dissatisfaction with the organisation of medical facilities in the Crimea, it was rumoured that Lord Panmure, the Secretary of War, had asked Professor Simpson to organise and take charge of a hospital staffed from Edinburgh,[25] but Simpson's involvement in the war effort was minimal. He did sponsor some of his young graduates to go out to the Crimea, and entrusted a case of chloroform to a Dr Dawson who was travelling to Constantinople. On arrival, Dawson established that the Sultan would not appreciate the gift, and decided to send it back to Simpson. He had it stowed aboard HMS *Agamemnon*, from whence it disappeared; 'and I have never seen it nor have I been able to obtain any clue of it since', Dawson later wrote plaintively to Simpson.[26]

Supplies were adequate at Scutari where it was used successfully for all operations, applied with a handkerchief held lightly to the face. Dr G. Pyemont Smith reported:

> The celebrated manifesto of Dr Hall against chloroform had not much attention paid to it at Scutari. I had been accustomed to the use of chloroform, but certainly had never seen it given to the extent that it was employed here. . . . Generally speaking, at Scutari, the patient was, by means of chloroform, brought into the condition of a dead body, and then it was not an operation, but a dissection that was performed.[27]

Even among those who used chloroform there was some confusion about its properties. A naval surgeon, George MacKay, reported that the first two amputations he performed were without chloroform, one because the limb was already virtually severed, the second because 'We had so much smoke and heated atmosphere from our lamps and candles and the smoke occasionally after gunpowder, that we did not deem it advisable to employ it until the action was nearly over'.[28] It seems that MacKay was under the mistaken impression that chloroform, like ether, was inflammable.

Dr George Macleod, who had studied medicine in Scotland during the exciting early years of anaesthesia, had few doubts about chloroform, and unlike Wrench, he had not been obliged to restrict its use.[29] After serving at Sebastopol he said that chloroform had been 'of inestimable value' in enabling prolonged examination of painful wounds, and producing the muscular relaxation essential to the easy removal of bullets: 'Then much is gained in field practice by the mere avoidance of the patient's screams when undergoing operation, as it frequently happens that but a thin partition, a blanket or a few planks, intervene between him who is being operated upon, and those who wait to undergo a like trial.' Having heard of the civilian use of chloroform to treat tetanus, Macleod tried it, but was forced to give it up. He recognised that it simply eased the symptoms, which returned when the treatment was withdrawn, and in the conditions of a field hospital, there were no assistants to spare for the prolonged administration.

In the 1855 edition of his book, seventy-year-old George James Guthrie showed that age need not be a bar to the acceptance of new ideas. Reports from the Crimea had shown that chloroform saved lives, and was no more harmful in gunshot wounds than any other injury. While his early pages advise caution,[30] the addendum, written after he had collected more information, especially on the major amputations, stated, 'The evidence . . . is sufficient to authorise surgeons to administer it in all such cases, with the expectation that it will always prove advantageous, an accidental death, such as has been observed from its use, being independent of the nature of the injury.'[31]

Six deaths had been attributed to its use, but all except one were cases of very severe injury. The exception was Pte Martin Kennedy, aged thirty-two, who had injured his finger when his musket went off accidentally. Seated in a chair, he received chloroform on a handkerchief for the amputation; just after the operation had commenced he suddenly expired.[32]

By October 1855 Dr Snow was reporting to the *Lancet* that the objections to chloroform had given way before further experience. While there was still some disagreement as to how to treat shock, Snow pointed out that after a gunshot wound, chloroform was preferable to the second shock of the knife.[33]

While British surgeons were arguing about the use of chloroform, French and Russian surgeons were using it with confidence. Charles Kidd, who believed that patients' emotions affected the way they took chloroform, described how the Russian surgeon Pirogoff had treated French prisoners in the hospital at Sebastopol and found they needed double or treble the amount of chloroform as did the calmer Russian soldier. The French, of course had just been taken prisoner, only to find their arms or legs were to be cut off by enemy surgeons, and were understandably in a state of some alarm.[34]

The experiences of French surgeons were universally favourable. Baudens reported in 1857 that in more than 30,000 administrations there had been no accidents from the use of chloroform throughout the war.[35] He believed that the calmness and tranquillity it conferred on the wounded assisted recovery. The Crimean experience put the seal on the almost complete acceptance of chloroform in France.

Following the end of hostilities in 1856 the Crimean Medical and Surgical Society was formed in London, and for six months held meetings to discuss what had been learnt during the war. Matters were made slightly awkward by the presence as chair of the newly elevated Sir John Hall. Surgeon James Mouat, who had earned a VC at Balaclava, opened the discussion on chloroform on 17 April. He supported Hall's 1854 memorandum as 'A wise and humane caution from an old and experienced officer in the field to his younger professional brethren'.[36]

Mouat, a man of the old school, thought that the mortality rate from chloroform was much higher than supposed. Provocatively, he suggested that medical men, not wanting the publicity that would follow after reporting a death from chloroform only recorded as such those that actually took place on the table. Many patients who had died twelve or twenty-four hours later were, he claimed, actually unacknowledged chloroform deaths. While not denying that chloroform was a boon to mankind, he concluded that in some states of shock chloroform could kill, and in minor surgery he recommended Dr Arnott's congelation as the safer course. His fellow surgeons were very much divided on both questions, with Dr Macleod strongly in opposition to Mouat. No guidelines emerged and it is probable that surgeons continued to do whatever they had been doing before.

In May 1857, anti-British feeling in India exploded into open revolt. White settlers – men, women and children – were killed in massacres and riots. The siege of Cawnpore in June and July ended in the death of 1,000 white residents. Meanwhile, at Lucknow, the British community found itself besieged in the British residency where both troops and civilians had taken refuge. They were under constant attack by shellfire and snipers, and medical resources were stretched. The senior civilian, Sir Henry Lawrence, suffered appalling wounds in the first assault. Examined under chloroform, his injuries were found to be inoperable. He was given opium for the pain, and when even that did not help, chloroform. He died two days later.[37] Some remnants of the old ideas were apparent. In July, Colonel Inglis's soldier servant, Vokins, was struck in the leg by roundshot. He was considered too weak to have chloroform, but able to endure amputation without anaesthetic, while his Colonel held him down.[38] He died seven weeks later. In August a young soldier called Studdy suffered the same fate. Judged unlikely to survive the depressant effects of chloroform, he was given a bottle of champagne before the operation, and was commendably brave throughout his ordeal, but died not long afterwards.[39] On 25 September, it seemed that relief was at hand. Sir Henry Havelock and Sir James Outram's Highlander regiments arrived, but they were not powerful enough a force to ensure the safety of the non-combatants in a break-out. They were obliged to stay and their presence put a further strain on supplies since they had brought none with them. Dr Fayrer, the senior medical man, had to eke out minimal stores of chloroform, and must have had some difficult decisions to make. Mrs Case, who had been widowed early in the attack, kept a daily diary and recorded that on 4 November a Mr Dashwood had been injured by roundshot, and both feet had been amputated, 'and as there is no chloroform, I fear he must have suffered a great deal'.[40] Seven days later, however, she records that Colonel Campbell had his leg amputated, and 'fortunately they were able to get some chloroform from Dr Fayrer'.[41]

No explanation is given of the sudden reappearance of chloroform, but it is tempting to suppose that Fayrer was saving it for those cases that needed it most. Campbell died the day after his operation. Eventually supplies were exhausted. According to Charles Kidd, surgeons at Lucknow compared survival rates for surgery with and without chloroform, and reported that the mortality from shock was far greater among those who did not have chloroform.[42] On 18 November, the arrival of Sir Colin Campbell's Highland Regiment enabled the survivors to leave Lucknow. Dashwood, who had survived the siege, died during the evacuation.

THE AMERICAN CIVIL WAR 1861–5

American surgeons had followed the events of the Crimea with great interest. When civil war erupted in 1861, and armies were mobilised and medical men engaged, chloroform was at once brought into use as the primary battlefield anaesthetic. It was usually given on a handkerchief or sponge. Since many operations were carried out in the open air, the open drop method was not used, as evaporation made it a lengthy and sometimes ineffective procedure, as well as highly wasteful.[43]

The South had considerable, though not insuperable, problems with supply. Lincoln's blockade, which became increasingly effective during the course of the war, often prevented supplies reaching the South, which did not have the manufacturing base of the North. As stocks dwindled, some ingenuity was required. Laboratories were established for drug manufacture, though these could not rival the Northern factories. Smuggling and blockade-running were vital sources, as was the capture of enemy stores. Some unscrupulous suppliers may have increased their profits by adulterating the product. One surgeon recalled using a supply of chloroform that smelled like turpentine.[44] (It was already known that turpentine had anaesthetic properties. In March 1861 a Dr Wilmshurst reported that when acting as a ship's surgeon his stock of chloroform had run out. He thought of trying turpentine and found it to be 'a very useful anaesthetic'.[45]) John Julian Chisholm, who had written a manual of military surgery for the Confederate Army, realised that apparatus could prevent evaporation of the scanty stocks and made use of a funnel as an inhaler. Later, he used a device shaped like a flattened cylinder. In one side was a perforated plate, and at the top, two nose pieces. These could be introduced into the nostrils while chloroform was dropped through the perforations on to a sponge or cloth inside.[46]

One of the most successful raiders of Union stocks was General Thomas Jonathan Jackson. He was nicknamed 'Stonewall' at the first battle of Bull Run in July 1861, though whether this was a compliment or not will never be known, as General Bee who so dubbed him was killed shortly afterwards. At the battle of Winchester in May 1862, Stonewall Jackson's Confederate Army routed the forces of Union General Banks, and seized enormous amounts of equipment and supplies, including medical wagons carrying 15,000 cases of chloroform. On 26 August, three days before the second battle of Bull Run, Jackson slipped behind the Union forces, and carried out a raid on the supply station at Manassas Junction, capturing what he could, which included many cases of chloroform, and destroying what couldn't be carried. Some months later, he had reason to be grateful. On 2 May 1863, after his victory at Chancellorsville, he carried out a night-time reconnoitre, and, returning in the dark, was mistakenly shot by his own men. His left arm was fractured, and it was decided to make an examination under chloroform. As the anaesthetic took effect, and the pain retreated, he exclaimed 'What an infinite blessing', and continued to murmur the word 'blessing' until he became insensible.[47] The examination confirmed that amputation was required, and this was carried out. Half an hour later, Jackson was conscious and able to have a cup of coffee. An hour later, he turned to Captain James Smith, who had been present at the operation, and asked if he had said anything under the chloroform. Smith reassured him that he had not. Jackson said, 'I have always thought it wrong to administer chloroform in cases where there is a probability of immediate death. It was the most delightful physical sensation I ever experienced. I seem to remember the most delightful music that ever greeted my ears, but I should dislike above all things to enter eternity in such a condition.'[48] Although he at first made good progress, complications set in, and Jackson died eight days later.

In the North, which had always, though not exclusively, favoured ether, there was concern about the use of chloroform, based on the by then antiquated idea that pain was an essential stimulant. There was no lack of support for this, as it was possible to trot out the authority of men like Porter and Cole, or quote the opinions of Guthrie and Velpeau expressed before chloroform earned their approval.[49]

Older surgeons had limited experience of anaesthesia, especially chloroform, and were concerned at the fatalities reported in the medical press, but it was the younger men who were on the battlefields, and they at once saw the advantages of chloroform. At the start of the war medical facilities were limited. Matters soon improved when the United States Sanitary Commission began a substantial distribution of supplies. Edward Squibb, founder of the drugs firm of E.R. Squibb and Co., had established efficient methods of mass production of ether and chloroform, and won the contract to supply the American forces. As in the South, administration of chloroform was by the simplest methods, on moistened lint or a sponge in a paper cone. The first inhalations were carried out at some distance from the patient's nose and mouth to allow dilution with air, and then the cloth was gradually advanced until anaesthesia was produced, when it was removed.[50]

Supplies were usually abundant, but there were occasional shortages, after Confederate capture of stores, or when the army had to abandon its wagons when making a rapid retreat. At Seven Pines in early June 1862, heavy use severely depleted stores, while at Glendale, later that month, hardly any was available, medical supplies being limited to what the hospital attendants could carry in their haversacks. On 27 June 1862, after the battle of Gaines Hill, heavy use and the abandonment of supplies meant that the chloroform ran out and essential surgery continued without it. In August 1862 at Richmond, Kentucky, Assistant Surgeon Irwin was taken prisoner, and was permitted to super-intend treatment of the wounded. There was a general lack of medical supplies and no chloroform for the twenty-seven major operations he had to perform.[51] After the battle of Perryville, in October 1862, Surgeon Hatchitt complained that supplies had not reached him and he had been forced to operate without chloroform, though he was able to replenish his supplies the following day.[52]

By 1864 the tide of the war had turned, and the reports of Union surgeons no longer mention any shortages. In 1865 Lincoln's blockade was preventing 50 per cent of supply ships getting through to the South, starving soldiers began to desert, and the Confederacy fell.

Southern surgeons reported only two chloroform deaths, but the most detailed statistics are those of the Union, in a six-volume study published after the war. The vast majority of operations were amputations. Another common operation was the repair of fistulas, anal fissures resulting from days in the saddle. Gangrene was a permanent concern. The standard treatment was to burn the tissues with nitric acid, a painful procedure, which chloroform made bearable. Northern surgeons used anaesthetics in about 80,000 instances. In only 8,900 cases was the nature of the anaesthetic used identified, and 76.2 per cent of these were under chloroform, with 14.7 per cent under ether, while in the remainder a mixture of chloroform and ether was used.[53] The use of ether, however, was effectively confined to general hospitals, while chloroform was almost always used in field hospitals. There were 254 reports of operations being carried out without anaesthetic, where no reason was given. After the battle of Iuka on 19 September 1862, for example, chloroform was not used in any of the operations, and 'not a groan or sign of pain was heard'.[54] If there had simply been a lack of supplies, the reporting surgeons would surely have mentioned this, so it is possible that concern about the complications of using chloroform in cases of gunshot wounds meant that chloroform was being withheld in certain cases.

Thirty-seven deaths were attributed to chloroform, four to ether, and two to the mixture.[55] Some accounts of these deaths are too sketchy for any conclusions to be drawn, but it is notable that about half do not relate to amputation of limbs, but are for the lesser procedures such as removal of toes and fingers, or extraction of bullets or bone fragments. Thirteen deaths are reported to have happened before the operation commenced, and fifteen reports comment on the suddenness of expiry, several surgeons describing the classic symptoms of cardiac arrest. The overall conclusion, however, was that the use of chloroform had greatly improved the survival rate in major operations. The official report was unequivocal:

> From the rapidity of its effects, and from the small quantity required – qualities which can only be appreciated at their proper values by the field surgeon when surrounded by hundreds of wounded anxiously awaiting speedy relief – chloroform was preferred by nearly all the field surgeons, and their testimony to its efficacy is almost unanimous, although all recommend the greatest care in its administration.[56]

There was one unusual proposal for the use of chloroform in the Civil War, that of a Mr Joseph Lott, who suggested using it to fill a hand-pumped fire engine and spraying it on enemy troops.[57] The importance of maintaining supplies for medicinal use and the known volatility of chloroform make it most unlikely that the idea ever came off the drawing board.

By the 1870s men of Sir John Hall's generation were no longer in control, and the young doctors who had survived the Crimea, India and the American Civil War had the authority of experience. Even the great champion of ether, H.J. Bigelow, grudgingly conceded that chloroform was better for army use. The argument about its suitability in military injuries was effectively over. Chloroform had gone to war – and it had won.

EIGHT

MURDER, MISHAP AND MELANCHOLY

> How can people who have been robbed be rendered instantly insensible? . . . We are still entirely sceptical, and so, we believe, is every one who knows anything about the matter; from this category we must, we fear, exclude most literary men, and the police altogether.
>
> *Editorial,* British Medical Journal, *1871*[1]

The enthusiasm of the medical profession for chloroform, and the rapidity with which it became a part of the Victorian scene, created a wholly unwarranted confidence in this most deadly anaesthetic, and encouraged a degree of misuse and carelessness that was frequently fatal. The first such casualty was Arthur Walker, an eighteen-year-old druggist's assistant of Aberdeen, who was so enamoured with the scent of the chloroform he weighed out that he used to sprinkle it on his handkerchief as cologne, and was often to be seen staggering drunkenly about the shop. His father, a foreman at the premises, tried unsuccessfully to dissuade him from this habit and was eventually obliged to hide the bottle. On 8 February 1848, Walker was in the warehouse, the only other employee present being a twelve-year-old boy. Discovering the chloroform bottle, Walker sprinkled some on a towel, which he laid on the counter, and leaned over it, inhaling the delicious vapour. Gradually the fumes overcame him and he sank forward, resting his head on his arms. The boy, knowing that Walker had been violent in the past when intoxicated, was more relieved than anything else to see him so quiet, and left him alone. When Walker's father arrived twenty minutes later, his son was dead. The *Scotsman*[2] loyally reported the medical opinion that since Walker had fallen face down on a moistened towel he had died not from the chloroform but from suffocation.[3]

Members of the general public found it relatively easy to obtain supplies of chloroform, which they inhaled for asthma, chronic painful complaints and insomnia. A common technique was to sprinkle a few drops on a handkerchief and retire to bed, placing the fragrant fabric over the face. Sometimes the relief was permanent, especially when the sufferer deliberately intensified the vapour by placing a hat or bedclothes over the head. A Mrs Mansell, who had been prescribed chloroform in 1856 for 'violent attacks of hysteria', found it produced such complete relief that she continued to use it frequently. During the next four years she developed a habit so alarming that both her husband and her doctor warned the local chemist not to supply her with any more. Despite this she was sold amounts of between five and fifteen ounces a day, which she would use an ounce at a time. The main safeguard against overdose was her ten-year-old daughter, who used to sprinkle the chloroform on the handkerchief and remove it when she judged that her mother had had sufficient. This system worked until the day when the little girl, romping with her playmates, was distracted by the game, and forgot to check on her mother until it was too late.[4]

There were, however, addicts who habitually inhaled enormous quantities of chloroform with apparent impunity. In 1892 James Bowskill, who described himself as a qualified chemist of London, was charged at Halifax with attempting to commit suicide by inhaling chloroform, attempted suicide being then a criminal offence.[5] Bowskill had been taken to the police station in a dazed condition and a piece of chloroform-soaked lint had been found in his pocket. He had earlier visited several chemists and obtained 4 ounces of chloroform. The case appeared proven, but before the magistrates' bench, Bowskill offered the perfect defence – he had not been trying to commit suicide at all, he was an addict. Questioned by the chairman, he successfully argued that the doses, which he said he took as stimulants, were not dangerous to him, and claimed that between Thursday and Friday he had inhaled 13½ ounces without injury. Bowskill further submitted that the police had failed to prove he had any intention of killing himself, adding that he had recently been charged with a similar offence at Huddersfield. Dismissing the main charge, the magistrates bound him over on his own recognisances of £20 to keep the peace for three months.

When chloroform was first introduced, doctors and dentists, pressed into adopting the new fashion, used it before they were entirely familiar with its properties. In January 1848, after a young lady had had a tooth extracted under chloroform, and departed well satisfied with the new 'painless principle', the surgeon and another gentlemen present were remarking on the pleasant odour of the anaesthetic. The surgeon was perhaps a little too appreciative of what remained on the handkerchief for he suddenly collapsed, and could not be revived for several minutes.[6] Dr Adams, resident physician to the Clyde Street Hospital, Glasgow, was less fortunate. Preparing to use chloroform, he inhaled it himself to try its strength, and not experiencing any serious result, tried it a second time, and fell back dead.[7]

Not everyone appreciated that chloroform was only poorly soluble in water. A Dr Sloman had been prescribing chloroform in a mixture for tetanus in 1849 and discovered, just in time to save his patient, that it tended to separate out and the bottle needed to be well shaken or the last dose would contain all the chloroform.[8]

As the century progressed and more complex surgical procedures became possible, it was not unusual for operations to continue long after dark, under the light of gas jets. This had the effect of accelerating the decomposition of chloroform, causing considerable distress to patients and medical staff as the theatre filled with poisonous fumes. The *British Medical Journal* was obliged to warn its readers about this in 1889.[9] In a Catholic hospital at Westphalia in 1898, a lengthy operation was required to a gunshot wound, and chloroform was administered for four hours. The two surgeons and the Sisters of Mercy were all overcome by the fumes, and one of the nurses died two days later.[10]

Some doctors were happy to prescribe chloroform for self-administration to trustworthy patients with chronic conditions, though Dr Snow[11] wisely diluted it with four parts of alcohol. One lady used two to three ounces of this mixture daily to relieve neuralgia. In 1884 a dentist's wife who used chloroform for just this purpose was incautious enough to take a bottle containing 8 ounces to bed with her. Having inhaled sufficient she was too woozy to replace the cork properly, and slept to her death on a chloroform-saturated pillow.[12]

Robert Ellis, whose complex inhaler had never really caught on, did not abandon his efforts to make chloroform inhalation safer. Lady Emily Childers, a friend of more than twenty-five years, took a keen interest in his work and even assisted with some of his experiments. She was, as Ellis explained in a long gloomy letter to *The Times* in 1875, a woman of temperate habits with a becoming caution about the consumption of medicines. When she began to suffer from a chronic painful complaint Ellis was confident that it was safe to prescribe chloroform, advising her to pour only ten or twenty drops at a time from the stock bottle into a small phial for inhalation. Ellis, whose researches should have taught him better, used a glass stopper for the stock bottle, not appreciating that the heat of a hand could induce sufficient evaporation to lift the stopper out of the bottle. Lady Childers's husband was fortunate to survive as he awoke one morning to find his wife dead beside him in a chloroform-soaked bed, the nearly empty stock bottle clutched in her hand, its stopper on the floor. It was no consolation to Ellis that the cause of the accident was proven when the stopper obligingly lifted out of the bottle during the inquest, causing a minor sensation in court.[13]

Occasionally, deaths occurred because the patient was given too free a hand in his or her own anaesthesia. It is hard to blame Mme Lebrune who, in 1849, having been instructed to hold the handkerchief at a distance, felt that she was not sufficiently 'under' for a tooth extraction; she pushed away the dentist's hand and pressed the handkerchief closely to her face, making several rapid inhalations. They were, unfortunately, her last.[14] There is rather less excuse for Dr Renwick of Alloa[15] and Dr Mailly of Mauritius[16] who both decided to administer chloroform to themselves during minor procedures in 1860 and 1861, and died rapidly.

In 1853 a lady was very fortunate to survive a forceps delivery in which her husband had been asked to hold a chloroformed handkerchief to her nose until she was insensible. He was so distracted by the proceedings that he left it in place too long and her heart and pulse ceased. Mouth-to-mouth resuscitation succeeded when all else had failed.[17]

CHLOROFORM ROBBERIES

It was not long after the introduction of chloroform that victims of robbery began claiming that they had been robbed while under its influence. There was usually little doubt that a crime had been committed, but the victim often reported no more than a brief exposure to some fragrant substance, which produced instant unconsciousness. Such claims were met with amused ridicule by the medical press, but the public, and that included juries, was all too willing to believe them. The dramatic evidence of a victim was often preferred to the sober expertise of a medical man, who knew that up to five minutes were required to anaesthetise even a willing subject. These claims may have been prompted by a wish to elevate the crime into something out of the commonplace, or to avoid admitting having been fooled into taking a drugged drink, or, in some cases, simply being drunk.

In 1850 Charlotte Wilson was alleged to have used chloroform for the theft of a hat and scarf from a man she had met in the street. At her trial, evidence was given that she passed a handkerchief lightly across his face, after which the pair entered a public house. Ten minutes and a glass or two of brandy later, the man collapsed, and Wilson was seen running away with his property.[18] The victim claimed he had been chloroformed, and the court believed him.

Mr Frederic Jewitt, a respectable young solicitor, had a particularly embarrassing situation to explain.[19] On 10 January 1850 he had been returning home from his office in Lime Street. Proceeding along Whitechapel High Road at nine o'clock he was supposedly accosted by a young woman who waved a handkerchief in his face. According to the virtuous Mr Jewitt, he had immediately become insensible, which explained why the following morning he awoke stark naked in a prostitute's bed in Thrawl Street, having been robbed of his money and valuables. Jewitt, who was reportedly very unwell after his ordeal, and failed to attend the trial of the two culprits, claimed that he had been chloroformed. His doctor was willing to say that chloroform might have been administered, but testified that when he called to see his patient Jewitt had clearly been under the influence of a narcotic, which must have been taken internally. The defendants did not deny the robbery and were transported for fifteen years.

There was profound scepticism regarding Jewitt's claims. Dr Snow pointed out that if unconsciousness had been instant and then lasted ten hours, chloroform could not have been used. Neither could he see how the crime had been committed as described in a busy thoroughfare without attracting attention: 'Persons who have been dead drunk are very unwilling to admit, even to themselves, that the result was the consequence of their own voluntary potations, and still less willing to admit it to the world, when they have to complain of having been robbed whilst in bad company.'[20]

Reading between those carefully phrased lines, the obvious conclusion was that the young solicitor had walked willingly to Thrawl Street on his own two feet, and been drugged when he got there.

Public concern about the use of chloroform in crime was such that in March 1851 an amendment was proposed to the Prevention of Offences Act, adding the following paragraph:

> And whereas it is expedient to make further provision for the punishment of persons using Chloroform, or other stupefying things, in order the better to enable them to commit felonies: be it enacted that if any person shall unlawfully apply or administer, to any other person any Chloroform, Laudanum or other stupefying or overpowering drug, matter or thing, with intent thereby to enable such offender or another person to commit any felony upon the person to whom the same may be applied or administered, or upon his or any other person's property, every such offender shall be guilty of felony, and being convicted thereof shall be liable, at the direction of the Court, to be transported for life, or for any term not less than seven years.[21]

Dr John Snow took exception to this and wrote a lengthy letter to Lord Campbell, Lord Chief Justice of the Court of the Queen's Bench, in which he described the reference to chloroform as 'alarming to the public, suggestive to the criminal, and little creditable to the sagacity and gravity of the law'.[22] Emphasising that it was impossible to chloroform an adult against his or her will, Snow said he knew of only two cases in which it had been used and in both it had led to the instant detection of the criminal.

On 13 October 1850 the Revd Mr Mackintosh, a clergyman in his seventies, was visiting Kendal in the Lake District to collect subscriptions to a charitable society, and had taken a room in a hotel. A scoundrel called Charles Venn had travelled on the same train, and was aware that the old man was carrying some gold sovereigns. There was no lock on the door of Mackintosh's room, so he wedged it shut with a chair and retired for the night, unaware that Venn had already concealed himself under the bed with a bottle of chloroform and a rag. Venn waited until midnight, when he was sure his victim was asleep, and then crawled out from under the bed; but the movement awoke the old man, who called out. He suddenly felt a cloth being pressed to his face, and despite his age put up a spirited resistance. A fierce fight ensued in which Venn, finding that chloroform was not as instant as the newspapers suggested, tried both battering and strangling the old gentleman, whose nightgown was soon spattered with blood. The tumult aroused the rest of the household, and the door was broken down. Venn, who tried unsuccessfully to convince the landlord that he had been sleepwalking, was immediately taken into custody. There was a smell of chloroform in the room, and the bottle was found under the bed and another in Venn's luggage. He was sentenced to eighteen months in prison with hard labour.[23]

Charles Jopling had been courting Mary Anne Elton, a virtuous twenty-year-old, for nine months, and in April 1850 they had attended a concert at a public house, which ended after midnight. Jopling was walking his sweetheart home when, overcome by amorous impulses, possibly fuelled by alcohol, he inveigled the trusting maiden into an alleyway and attempted to take liberties which she strongly resisted. Jopling must have been prepared for this reaction for he suddenly produced a handkerchief, which he soaked from a phial of chloroform and attempted to apply to her face. Mary pushed this aside and fled, crying out for a policeman. Fortunately, a constable was nearby and immediately came running to help. Jopling, after begging her not to press charges, ungallantly claimed that Mary was lying and tried to throw away the incriminating evidence, but the constable apprehended not only Jopling but the handkerchief and phial. Protestations of innocence in the magistrate's court rang hollow in the face of medical evidence that chloroform had been detected on the exhibits. The case was adjourned for a week but at the next hearing Mary said she no longer wished to prosecute and pleaded instead for mercy – she had married Jopling the day before. The slightly bemused magistrate let him off with a stern lecture.[24]

In citing these cases Snow was perhaps being naive and it is not surprising that his plea was respectfully declined. He did not for example consider a weak or a drunken victim, or that there might be more than one assailant, as in the case of the unfortunate Mrs Savage of Ulverston. That lady was walking home in June of 1857 with a bundle of clothing she had recently purchased when she was set upon by three men and a woman, who stole not only her bundle and her purse, but every stitch she was wearing. She was obliged to cower behind some bushes until she was able to attract the attention of some passing females. Her claim that she had been chloroformed has more to commend it than most, as she would have been easily overpowered, and only brief unconsciousness was required.[25]

John W.R. McIntyre, who analysed the field in 1988, concluded that, while it is possible to administer chloroform to a conscious and unwilling subject, this can only be done by exercising considerable violence, and is a hazardous activity which may well end in the death of the victim. If the administrator intends not murder, but prolonged unconsciousness for the purposes of robbery or rape, it is not sufficient simply to render the victim unconscious – the administration needs to be constantly and carefully maintained, and some skill is required. A large initial dose is more likely to end in death than lengthy unconsciousness.[26]

In July 1854 chloroform was part of the armoury of John Carden of Tipperary, a 43-year-old landowner, who, with the aid of some armed men, attempted to carry off Miss Eleanor Arbuthnot, an heiress less than half his age who had rejected his offers of marriage.[27] One Sunday, as Eleanor was about to drive away from church in a carriage, Carden rode up, the traces were cut, and the coachman held at knifepoint. The other three occupants of the carriage were Eleanor's older sister Laura, her married and pregnant sister Mrs George, and a lady friend, Miss Lyndon. Carden must have thought it would be a simple matter of opening the door and pulling Eleanor out, while the ladies screamed and reached for their smelling-salts. Instead, he was met with fierce resistance from Miss Lyndon who punched him in the face and gave him a bloody nose. He was able to drag Miss Lyndon from the carriage, and Mrs George very sensibly got out, these two ladies immediately running for assistance. Carden then pulled Laura out, but she clung to him like a limpet and they both ended up rolling on the ground, Carden yelling for help to an associate, who eventually pulled Laura off him. Carden then dashed back to the carriage where Eleanor was resisting the attempt of another of his men to pull her out by holding on to a strap. Laura jumped up and ran after Carden, hitting him over the head. When the strap broke, she helped her sister, who was half out of the carriage, and Eleanor managed to regain her position, and, wedging herself in place with one foot, kicked Carden repeatedly in the chest with the other, while he made earnest protestations of love. Meanwhile, help had arrived, and Carden and his ruffians fled but were soon captured. Among the items he had laid aside in preparation for the proposed flight and forced marriage were two bottles of chloroform.

Carden later claimed he had been concerned lest the abduction would cause hysterics, and shortly before the attempt he had consulted his physician, Dr Forsyth, as to the best thing to give a lady prone to hysteria. Forsyth advised ten to twenty drops of chloroform in water, or it could be given by inhalation, and he rolled up his handkerchief to demonstrate. He supplied Carden with a small bottle, and when Carden commented that he was concerned lest the bottle break, obligingly gave him another one. Carden claimed he had first tried out the remedy on himself and, while finding it an effective sedative, it gave him a headache and made him feel sick, so he decided not to use it. At the trial in July, Dr Forsyth was given a tough time by the Attorney General:[28]

Attorney General: You did not ask for whom he intended these things?
Forsyth: I did not . . . I formed no idea about it. I did not wish to pry into any matter of the kind.
Attorney General: What did you mean by that? Had you any suspicion?
Forsyth: Not the most remote.
Attorney General: Then why did you use the word 'pry'?
Forsyth: From his position and rank in society, I did not wish to ask questions.
Attorney General: You thought his rank entitled him to administer drugs to a lady?
Forsyth: No.

Carden was sentenced to two years' imprisonment with hard labour, but earned the sympathy of the public, who felt that he was a dashing fellow, and Miss Arbuthnot a minx who should have accepted him.

Public willingness to accept tales of chloroform crime seems not to have abated. In 1975 the *Sunday Times* reported the claim of railway officials that passengers in the Orient Express were being robbed of valuables as they slept after thieves sprayed chloroform into the carriages.[29] McIntyre's comment on a similar technique said to have been used in a rape case is that even in a small bedroom 1,000 ml would have had to be sprayed and vaporised to render an occupant insensible to sensory stimuli.[30] One can only speculate on the quantities required for a sleeping-carriage.

SUICIDE

The first recorded suicide with chloroform took place in 1851, in Vienna.[31] The chief physician of the Royal Hospital, Dr Reyer, apparently in good health and spirits, was one day conversing with his colleagues on the apparently academic subject of the least painful form of death. He must have come to a satisfactory conclusion, for later the same evening he was found dead in his room, having fastened a bladder filled with chloroform round his mouth and nostrils with adhesive plaster.

While it was all too easy to die from inhaled chloroform, when the fluid was taken by mouth, it proved to be a dubious means of committing suicide. Consumed in quantity, it was often vomited up, so not all of it was absorbed, and it was not invariably fatal. One Friday in 1851, a young man walked into a barber's shop at 2 p.m., sat down and appeared to fall asleep. No notice was taken of him for two hours, after which it was found that he could not be roused and a surgeon was sent for. He was taken to hospital comatose, and a stomach pump was used, but by 11 p.m. his pulse was slow, his skin pale and cold, and he was breathing stertorously, with froth being expelled convulsively from his mouth. Over the next few days, however, he slowly recovered and on the Tuesday he was well enough to go home. He said he had drunk 4 ounces of chloroform at 1 p.m., and had no recollection of going into the barber's shop.[32]

When chloroform was fatal, death could take hours or even days. Many suicides, possibly thinking that they would peacefully sleep themselves to death, found that their lingering demise was actually due to the damage done to the lining of the stomach. In 1858 a Dr Bain was called to a patient to find her unconscious, and saw a nearly empty 3-oz chloroform bottle beside her.[33] He used a stomach pump, and after several hours during which her respiration failed and restarted a number of times, she recovered consciousness and admitted that she had drunk the chloroform following some domestic unpleasantness. The narcotic effect eventually wore off, but despite every effort to mitigate the corrosive effects of the chloroform on her stomach she suffered for another seven days and died.

Another protracted and unpleasant death was that of Dr Robert Mortimer Glover whose career had not prospered since the inquest on Hannah Greener.[34] He had left Newcastle for London in 1854, and worked at the Royal Free Hospital, but was formally reprimanded in the following year for neglecting his patients and failing to obtain his Licence of the Royal College of Physicians. Soon afterwards, Glover joined the army medical corps and departed England to serve at Scutari in the Crimea. While there he contracted amoebic dysentery, an affliction for which he blamed many of his later woes, as he began to take opium and chloroform for relief, sometimes in excessive amounts. He formally resigned from the Royal Free in 1856 and his main professional activity was writing medical pamphlets. His once promising career was in ruins. He relied on former colleagues for financial support and also lodged with Walter Mingay Rochfort, a chemist, who has been suspected of practising medicine illegally using Glover's name. It was probably Rochfort who supplied him with the drugs he was taking, often to the point of insensibility. By 1859 his behaviour was becoming so erratic that his friends were anxious for his health and sanity.

On 10 March 1859 Glover, then forty-two, married 36-year-old Maria Matilda Sarah Hickson. How the couple met is not known. Two years previously Maria had been living in the St Marylebone workhouse, where she made a living as a needlewoman. Maria had a long history of mental instability, and had previously been confined to an asylum in Northumberland, In 1857 she was transferred to Colney Hatch lunatic asylum with attacks of violent mania, during which she attempted to bite her attendants.[35] Somehow, Maria managed to escape. Shortly before the match Glover approached an old friend for the loan of £1 with which to finance the honeymoon. It was with some distress that his friends saw him marry someone who was 'as much a lunatic as himself' but there was little they could do.[36] The couple lived in a hotel for a week before Maria was recaptured, and returned to Colney Hatch. She was transferred to a Newcastle asylum in 1872.

On the evening of 8 April, Glover was visited by Frederick Gant, who had been a colleague of his at the Royal Free and had also served in the Crimea. They discussed an article in the *Lancet*, then Glover referred briefly to his marriage describing it as 'a bad affair', though he did not seem to be depressed. After a while, Glover left the house asking Gant to stay till his return, which was in twenty minutes. The two men continued to talk, mainly about their Crimean experiences, but during the course of the conversation Glover inexplicably left the room and returned a number of times at about five-minute intervals. So curious was this behaviour that Gant asked him if anything was the matter, but Glover replied that he had never been in better health. He suddenly appeared to be intoxicated, muttered incoherently and collapsed, snoring loudly. He had hardly any pulse, his pupils were contracted and his face was pale and sweaty. Gant tried to revive him, and at that moment Rochfort arrived and at once identified the smell of chloroform. A galvanic battery and ammonia were used to try and revive the patient, who was too weak for emetics, and when Gant left at 1 a.m. Glover was sleeping 'as I have seen him on other occasions when under the influence of alcohol, camphor or opium, taken immoderately as was his habit, to induce anaesthesia'.[37]

Four hours later Rochfort sent for another doctor and by 9 a.m. Glover was able to swallow an emetic. After an hour and a half he vomited about half a gallon of brownish blood and mucus smelling strongly of chloroform, and an hour later purged copious quantities of a similar liquid. Friction, hot flannels and galvanism were applied, but despite all efforts he became increasingly feeble and died at 8 p.m.[38]

It was Gant's belief that Glover had swallowed at least 5 ounces of chloroform, and few people should have known better that Glover the effect of such a dose. Unsurprisingly the *Daily Telegraph* anticipated the inquest verdict by announcing Glover's 'melancholy suicide'[39] but after evidence was given of Glover's habitual use of narcotics, and his brother William stated that the deceased was opposed to suicide, the inquest jury returned the verdict that he had swallowed the chloroform as an intoxicant, and not with any intention of injuring himself or destroying life.

PROSECUTIONS

Given the numbers of deaths under chloroform it is surprising that so few doctors were ever prosecuted for negligence. The English journals reported these cases and issued grave words of warning to doctors, but it is noticeable that successful prosecutions did not for the most part happen in the British Isles.

In 1852 the *Lancet* reported the death of a lady in Strasbourg. She had been so terrified of the dentist that she had tried to run away, but had been persuaded back. More afraid of the pain than she was of the chloroform, she submitted to the anaesthetic in a state of great anxiety. The teeth were successfully extracted, but the lady was found to be dead. It was suggested that the administrator had been negligent, and the matter was brought before the courts. Dr Sédillot gave evidence that the anaesthetist had used an accepted mode of administration, and there was an immediate acquittal.[40]

In 1853 a surgeon and his assistant were tried in Paris after the death of a 24-year-old man under chloroform, the operation being the removal of a tumour from his cheek.[41] It was claimed that the room was not sufficiently ventilated, they had used chloroform unnecessarily and had not taken any precautions in case of accident. They were found guilty of 'homicide by imprudence' and fined the equivalent of £2.

In Ireland in 1873 a Mr Lambe, a tall, powerful 32-year-old, requiring amputation of some injured toes, died under chloroform, and his widow, claiming negligence, sued two doctors at Wicklow assizes, demanding £1,000 in damages. There was no post-mortem, but Lambe's doctor gave evidence that he was a man of nervous temperament, occasionally given to fainting, which supported the defendants' case that the patient had died from a heart defect impossible to detect in life. The court was in agreement and they were acquitted.[42] The *Lancet*, exhibiting some anxiety for the risks run by surgeons, pointed out that in the current state of knowledge, any medical man might be taken to court and have witnesses state that ether should have been given as it was less dangerous: 'Medical opinion has become unsettled upon this point, and it is of paramount importance that some definite decision should be arrived at.'

American courts, especially in the mainly ether-using Northern states, were less inclined than their British counterparts to agree that chloroform deaths were an unavoidable accident. A practitioner who used chloroform had to be seen to take every precaution and, if the patient died, had to assume some responsibility. In Philadelphia in 1878, there was a death after chloroform was administered by a dentist. A jury of medical men was empanelled by a coroner who was also a medical practitioner and they returned a verdict charging him with 'criminal ignorance in administering so powerful a remedy not having made any examination of the patient'.[43] He was committed to prison without bail and ultimately appeared before a grand jury where he was found guilty, although his sentence is not recorded.

In Australia, too, a chloroform death could be seen as the fault of the administrator. In Sydney in 1888 the husband of a lady who had died under chloroform took action for damages and was awarded £200.[44]

Contrast this with the case of *Rex v. Lancaster and Crook* at Liverpool Assizes in February 1902.[45] The defendants were not qualified dentists but practised as 'teeth extractors', and gave chloroform before operating. A lady patient who had been operated on before was given chloroform on a handkerchief and did not regain consciousness. Having no idea what to do about this, they made no attempt at resuscitation but raised her into a sitting position and ran for a doctor, who could do nothing except pronounce the woman dead. It was pointed out at the trial that the men had successfully given chloroform 350 times previously, and there was no evidence that the woman had died of an overdose. As long as they didn't call themselves dentists, their practice was perfectly legal, and there was no law to prevent them administering chloroform. The judge formally directed an acquittal.

MURDER

Given the pungent smell and strong taste of chloroform it seems like an unpromising material with which to commit a murder by persuading the victim to drink it, yet there are several cases on record, two of them notorious, the following one virtually unknown.[46]

Winifred Markland was twenty-seven, and, by the standards of the day, not of good character. Though unmarried she had two years previously given birth to a stillborn child. According to the custom of the time, her father had turned her out of the family home in Stockport, and she lived in nearby Manchester where she sometimes styled herself as a widow, or a married woman whose husband had gone to America. Winifred earned her living as a sewing-machine worker, but in the slack season she was not averse to supplementing her income by entertaining gentlemen who would give her presents of money. She shared lodgings with Fanny Stevenson, a respectable hat maker who preferred to turn a blind eye to Winifred's slack-season activities. Late in September 1876, Winifred had been away from home for a few days visiting a gentleman in Runcorn, some thirty miles away, and on Monday 2 October she returned, saying that she expected the Runcorn gentlemen to visit her at 10 p.m. that night. Winifred was in buoyant spirits saying that the gentleman had given her £1 and would give her £2 that evening. Fanny, who was in no doubt about the nature of the 'visit', asked Winifred if she was not concerned that she would get into trouble, but Winifred said no, she would see to it. This conversation would not have been unusual except for the identity of the gentleman in question, for he was none other than Father Joseph Daly, a 37-year-old Roman Catholic priest who had charge of the chapel at Runcorn. Fanny preferred not to be at home when Winifred was 'entertaining' and left to spend the night with her sister. When she departed, Winifred was very much alive, and looking forward to receiving her visitor.

That evening, promptly at 10 p.m., a gentleman knocked on the door of Winifred's lodgings. Ada Purdie, who lived nearby, observed Winifred open the door to admit the visitor and later described him as tall and stout with whiskers, a portrait sufficiently similar to the appearance of Father Daly that it was never challenged. Mary Ann Ogden, who lived across the road, knew Father Daly by sight and had seen him visit Winifred before. She was convinced that the man she saw enter the house was the priest. On the following day, Fanny returned home, but to her surprise found the front door locked and was obliged to borrow a spare key from a neighbour. Winifred was obviously at home, for glancing through the open bedroom door Fanny saw her friend's arm hanging out of the side of the bed. It was not the side on which Winifred usually lay, and Fanny, assuming Winifred had someone in bed with her, did not enter the room. Shortly afterwards, Fanny went out, and when she returned at 2 p.m. nothing had changed. Still nothing struck her as unusual, and she later went out again and spent the night at a friend's house. The following morning, however, when she returned to find Winifred still in the same position, and decomposition setting in, she realised that something was wrong. A doctor and a policeman were called, and they examined and removed for testing some bottles and glasses found beside the bed, while the body was sent for post-mortem.

The inquest was held on 26 October; by then the tests had revealed that the bottles and glasses found at Winifred's bedside contained nothing more than the then-popular concoction of gin, water and sugar. The doctor appeared and declared that Winfred had died of alcoholic poisoning. A chemist then gave evidence to say that he had analysed the stomach contents and found, apart from the gin, water and sugar, 48 grains of chloroform, a sufficient quantity to show that the deceased had swallowed a fatal dose. He had also carried out tests for the constituents of chlorodyne and had found none. His conclusion was that Winifred had died from drinking liquid chloroform. The coroner recalled the doctor, who was asked if he wanted to reconsider his opinion as to the cause of death, and unsurprisingly he did. There had been no chloroform in the house before the death, and there was none in it afterwards. The conclusion was obvious – someone had arrived with a bottle of chloroform, persuaded Winifred to drink some, and had departed with the incriminating bottle. There was only one candidate for that role and he was Father Joseph Daly.

Winifred's aggrieved father, mill-worker John Markland, took the stand. He was unrepentant at having thrown her out of his house, and said he had often spoken to her about her imprudent and thoughtless behaviour. He had disapproved of her association with Father Daly, and had even remonstrated with the priest on one occasion as he felt there had been improper liberties. After the evidence of Ada Purdie and Mary Ann Ogden, things looked extremely serious for Father Daly, but that gentleman, far from being defensive about his role in the matter, demanded to be sworn in as a witness, and took the stand with confidence. The coroner having observed that there was some suspicion against him, Daly stated that he could prove his innocence. He declared the accusations to be scandalous, and denied absolutely that he was the father of Winifred's child or that there had ever been anything improper between them. Moreover, he could show conclusively that he was nowhere near the house on the night of Winifred's death. He then produced three witnesses, all of whom knew him by sight, all of whom gave him an unimpeachable alibi. A booking clerk at Runcorn station had seen him at half past nine, at which hour it would have been impossible for him to have travelled to Manchester in time to be on Winifred's doorstep at ten. A hotel-keeper had seen Father Daly in Runcorn shortly before 10 o'clock and an auctioneer had seen him at about the same time. Daly denied that he had ever agreed to visit Winifred that evening. Charged with the fact that she had said so, he commented regretfully that the deceased had not been a truthful person.

Daly freely admitted that, on hearing that there was suspicion against him, he had gone to Runcorn and asked people he had met that night to give evidence that they had seen him, but said it was natural that he should do so to defend his reputation. The coroner summed up. He found that there was no evidence that Winifred had committed suicide and the absence of the chloroform bottle was a strong suggestion that she had been murdered. No mention was made of the difficulty of inducing Winifred to drink the chloroform and it must simply have been assumed that the murderer had achieved this by first making her drunk. The jury duly delivered the verdict that Winifred had been wilfully murdered, but there was insufficient evidence to say by whom. Father Daly left the court without a stain on his character, and there the matter rested. No one was ever brought to trial and the case is officially unsolved.

Just over two months later, however, Father Daly was in court again, but this time at the Knutsford quarter sessions and he was in the dock.[47] While this case has nothing to do with chloroform it does throw some further light on the character of the priest, and conclusions may be drawn about his innocence or guilt of Winifred Markland's murder. When he arrived in Runcorn the previous June, Daly had for the first few weeks lodged with one of his parishioners, William Hailwood, a grocer. During his stay, he had commenced an improper relationship with Hailwood's eighteen-year-old daughter, who was also called Winifred, and two days after he had secured his own lodgings he seduced her. Daly's frequent visits to Winifred were noted with disapproval by Hailwood's 22-year-old son. William junior had informed Father Daly that he was not to visit the house again unless he and his father were present, but this had been ignored. Notes had been passed between the couple, and visits made during which Daly had been supposedly sleeping in a spare room but had actually shared young Winifred's bed. Daly, who had said he was short of money for bills, had inveigled Winifred into giving him the key to the room where the shop takings were kept and she had brought him a piece of iron to break open the money drawer. The two had tried to make it look like a burglary but so unsuccessfully that the police at once suspected the thief was a member of the household, and it seemed as if suspicion might fall on young William. Winifred confessed the crime to her cousin, and was eventually persuaded to tell all. Hailwood whipped his convent-educated daughter and turned her out of the house, and Father Daly found himself in court accused of the theft of £12.

Winifred's testimony caused a sensation. Daly, who asked to be seated, as he claimed he was unwell, could only claim that Miss Hailwood was not telling the truth, but there was corroborative evidence from the servants of notes passed and he was found guilty and sentenced to eighteen months' imprisonment with hard labour. The day after reporting the verdict, the *Manchester Guardian*, without referring to the case in any way, published a paragraph from the *Lancet* warning professional men to take great care in their dealings with females especially if young and unmarried because of the dangers of delusional accusations by hysterical and neurotic women against men of unsullied reputation. So was the Revd Father Joseph Daly an unfortunate and much maligned man, or was he a scoundrel who was extremely lucky to get away with murder?

The *Lancet*'s comments highlight a common dichotomy with chloroform-related crimes. In cases such as Mr Jewitt's, no one doubted that he had been robbed, the only question being whether chloroform was involved. There was another circumstance, however, where it was extremely difficult to prove that any crime had taken place, and this was when women accused doctors or dentists of improper conduct. Opinion, as one might expect, was very firmly on the side of the professional gentlemen.

NINE

INNOCENT WOMEN

I am going to gaol with joy unspeakable.

W.T. Stead[1]

In February 1848 a doctor wrote to Professor James Simpson to express a very particular concern. He felt that there should be more legislation about the sale of chloroform to the public, and predicted that it was sure to be used to debauch innocent women.[2] He was right – but how right it is impossible to determine.

Studies of Victorian prostitution have shown that some of the girls were introduced into that way of life by being tricked into believing they were destined either for respectable work or even marriage, and once in the hands of the procurers they were then drugged and violated. Chloroform was certainly one of the drugs used. The girls rarely protested afterwards, as they usually did not know the identity of their assailant, and a woman who had lost her chastity was seen as a discredited witness.

When chloroform was first introduced it suited its enthusiasts to deny that it produced erotic sensations, but the tune changed dramatically when patients began to accuse surgeons of sexual assault. Doctors and dentists in private practice, lacking any assistance, habitually administered chloroform to patients when no other person was present. This was medically highly unsatisfactory, as the journals frequently pointed out, since a practitioner could not adequately monitor the condition of his anaesthetised patient and perform surgery at the same time. Such a practice also exposed the professional man to accusations of criminal behaviour. It was officially assumed that he was always innocent.

Stories were common in the medical journals of ladies displaying amorous behaviour towards their surgeons when

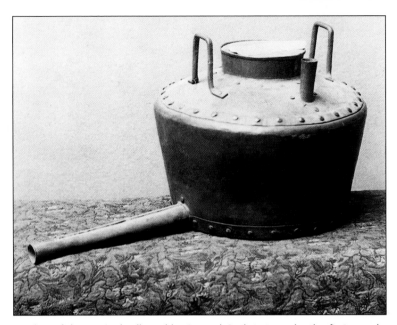

Replica of the original still used by Samuel Guthrie to make the first sample of chloroform in 1831. (*By kind permission of the Jefferson County Historical Society, Watertown, NY, USA*)

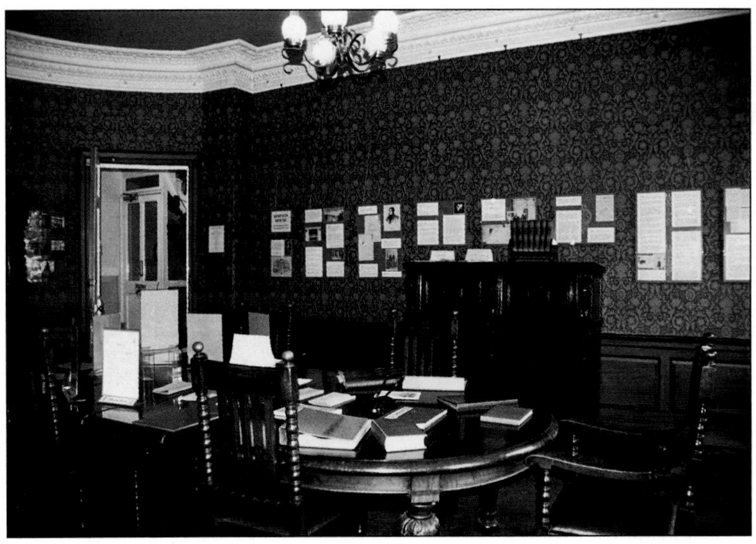

The 'Discovery Room' where experiments first revealed the anaesthetic power of pure chloroform, 52 Queen Street, Edinburgh. (*Author's collection. Photographed by kind permission of Simpson House*)

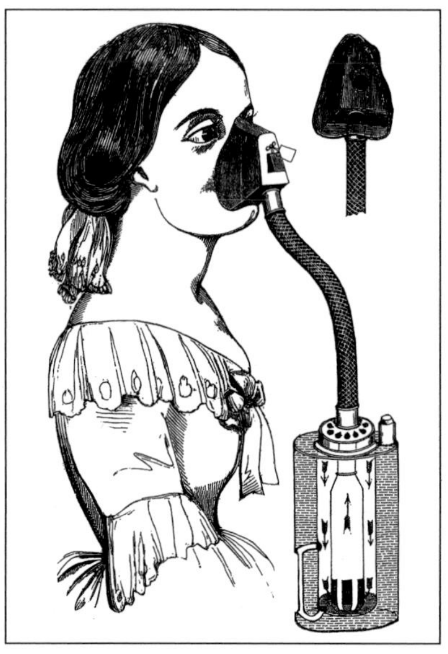

Dr John Snow's chloroform inhaler. (*By kind permission of the British Library. Shelfmark 7460.d.36*)

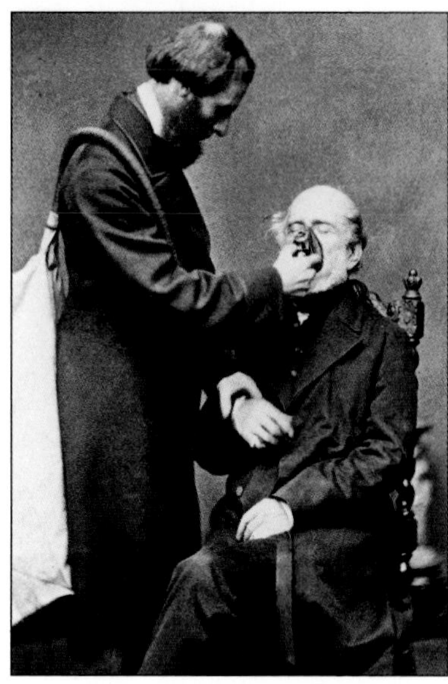

Dr Clover and his apparatus. (*By kind permission of the Nuffield Department of Anaesthetics, John Radcliffe Infirmary, Oxford*)

1015 1016 1020

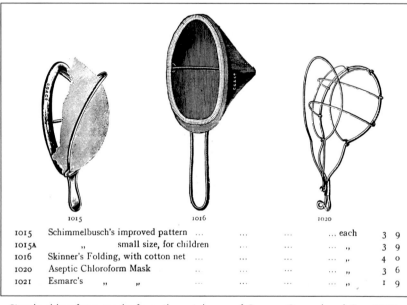

1015	Schimmelbusch's improved pattern	each	3	9
1015A	" small size, for children	"	3	9
1016	Skinner's Folding, with cotton net	"	4	0
1020	Aseptic Chloroform Mask	"	3	6
1021	Esmarc's " "	"	1	9

Simple chloroform masks from the catalogue of Cuxson Gerrard and Co., 1910. (*By kind permission of Cuxson Gerrard and Co.*)

Thursday 7 April

Administered Chloroform to the Queen in her confinement. Slight pains had been experienced since Sunday. Dr Locock was sent for about nine o'clock this morning, stronger pains having commenced, and he found the os uteri had commenced to dilate a very little. I received a note from Sir James Clark a little after ten asking me to go to the Palace. I remained in an apartment near that of the Queen along with Sir J. Clark Dr Ferguson and (for the most part of the time) Dr Locock till a little after twelve. At a thirty minutes past twelve by a clock in the Queen's apartment I commenced to give a little chloroform with each pain, by pouring about 15 minims by measure on a folded handkerchief. The first stage of labour was nearly over when the chloroform was commenced. Her Majesty expressed great relief from the application, the pain being very trifling during the uterine contractions, and whilst between the periods of contraction there was complete ease. The effect of the chloroform was not at any time carried to the extent of quite removing consciousness. Dr Locock thought the chloroform prolonged the intervals between the pains, and retarded the labour somewhat. The infant was born at 13 minutes past one by the clock in the room (which was 3 minutes before the right time) consequently the chloroform was inhaled for 53 minutes. The placenta was expelled in a very few minutes, and the Queen appeared very cheerful and well, expressing herself much gratified with the effect of the chloroform.

Entry in Dr John Snow's notebook, 7 April 1854, recording his administration of chloroform to Queen Victoria. (*By kind permission of the Royal College of Physicians, London*)

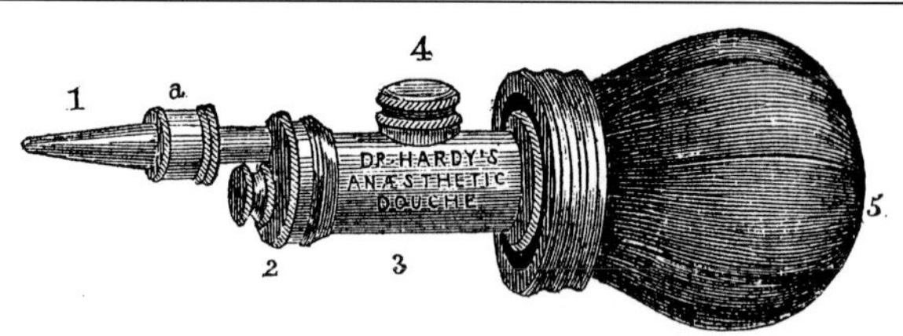

1, small pipe containing a valve *(a)* for transmitting the vapour; 2, air-valve; 3, chamber containing within it a sponge for holding the chloroform; 4, screw stopper for closing sponge-chamber; 5, India-rubber bottle attached.

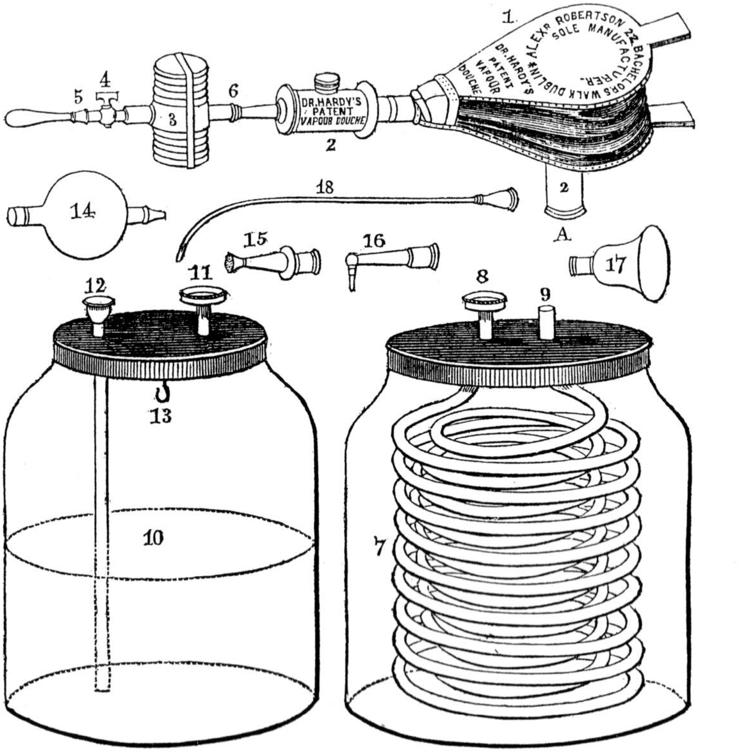

1, bellows; 2: 2, sponge-chambers; 3, elastic chamber; 4, stop-cock; 5 and 6, connecting screws; 7, jar; 8, connecting screw of spiral tube for attaching it to sponge-chamber at A; 9, end of spiral tube: 10, jar; 11, tube to connect to chamber 2 at A: 12, air-tube; 13, hook for thermometer; 14, glass or platinum chamber; 15, 16, 17, various conveyance pipes for attaching to screws 5 or 6: 18, catheter.

Dr Hardy's patented chloroform douches, 1854. The upper is designed to give short puffs of vapour, the lower to give a stronger continuous stream. (*By kind permission of the British Library. Shelfmark PP.3190*)

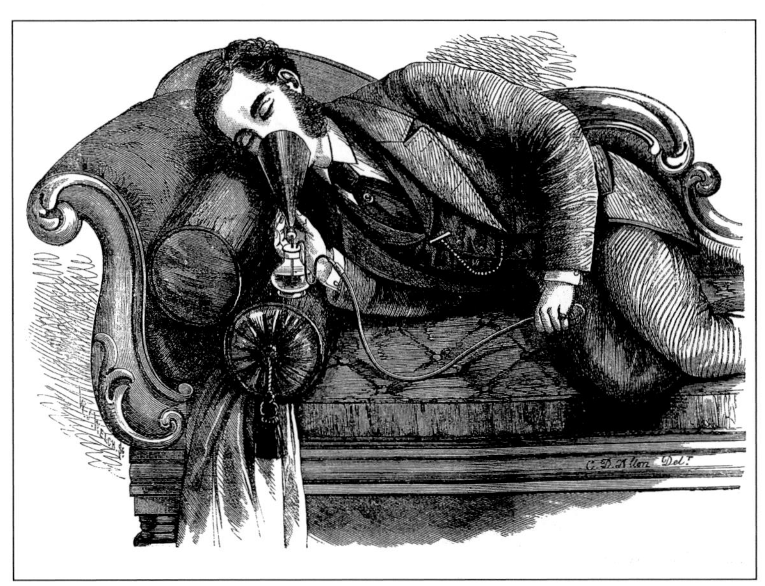

Dr John Mann Crombie's patented apparatus for the self-administration of chloroform, 1873. (*By kind permission of the British Library. Shelfmark 7462.bb.46*)

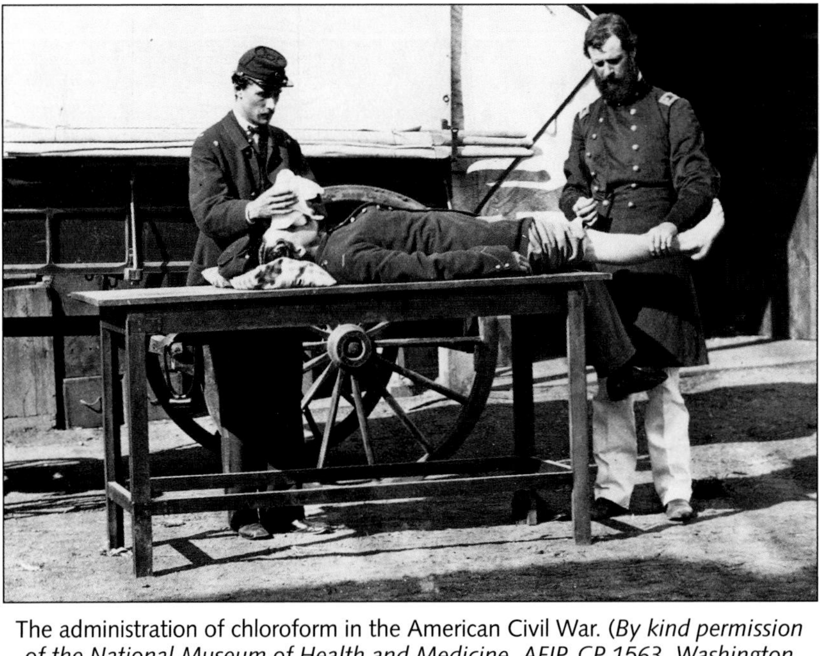

The administration of chloroform in the American Civil War. (*By kind permission of the National Museum of Health and Medicine, AFIP, CP 1563, Washington DC, USA*)

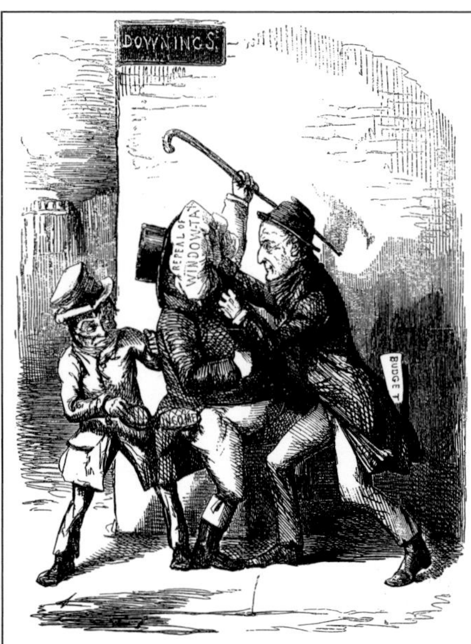
DOWNINGS
REPEAL OF WINDOW-TAX
BUDGET
DARING ROBBERY OF AN OLD GENTLEMAN NAMED "BULL,"
By the Aid of Chloroform.

Robbery under chloroform, as seen by *Punch*, 1851. (*By kind permission of the British Library. Shelfmark LD34*)

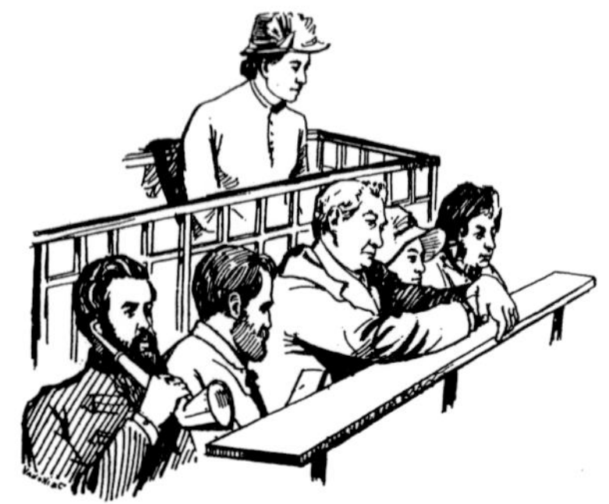

THE

ELIZA ARMSTRONG CASE:

BEING A VERBATIM REPORT

OF THE

PROCEEDINGS AT BOW STREET.

WITH

MR. STEAD'S SUPPRESSED DEFENCE.

WITH ILLUSTRATIONS.

"PALL MALL GAZETTE" OFFICE, 2, NORTHUMBERLAND STREET, STRAND, LONDON, W.C.

1885.

The defendants in the Eliza Armstrong case. Mrs Jarrett in the witness box, and from left to right, W. Bramwell Booth, W.T. Stead, Samson Jacques, Mrs Combe, Mme Mourey.

Resuscitation after chloroform accident. Method of H.A. Kelly, gynaecological department at Johns Hopkins University, 1892. (*By kind permission of the British Library. Shelfmark Ac.3831*)

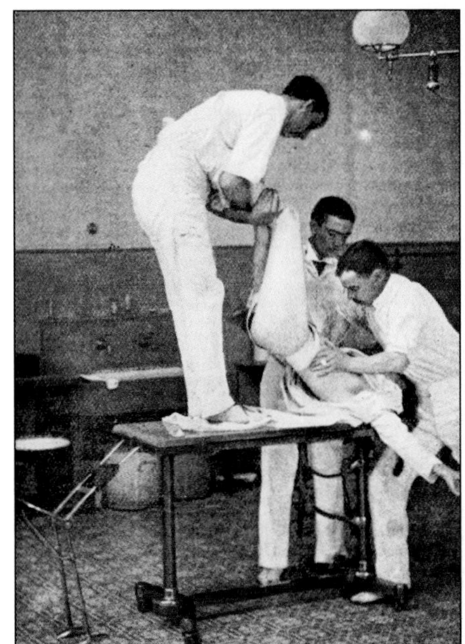

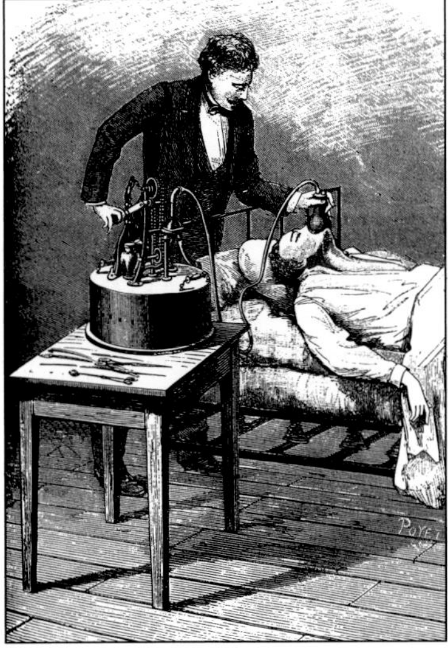

The anaesthetising machine of Raphäel Dubois, *c.* 1891.

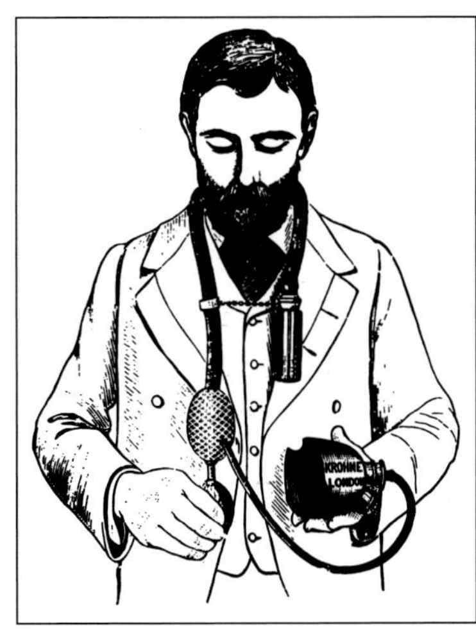

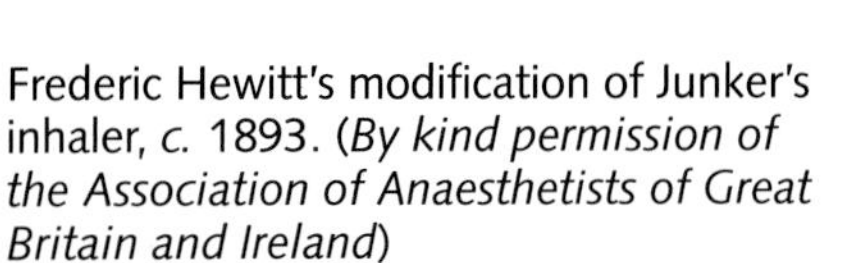
Frederic Hewitt's modification of Junker's inhaler, *c.* 1893. (*By kind permission of the Association of Anaesthetists of Great Britain and Ireland*)

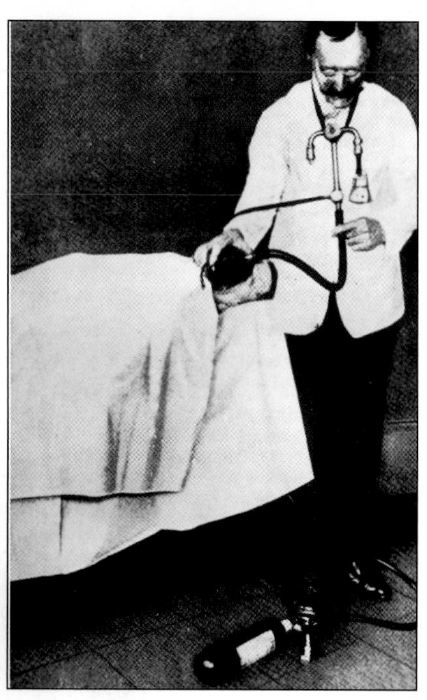

The Vernon Harcourt inhaler in use, with added oxygen, 1914. (*By kind permission of the Association of Anaesthetists of Great Britain and Ireland*)

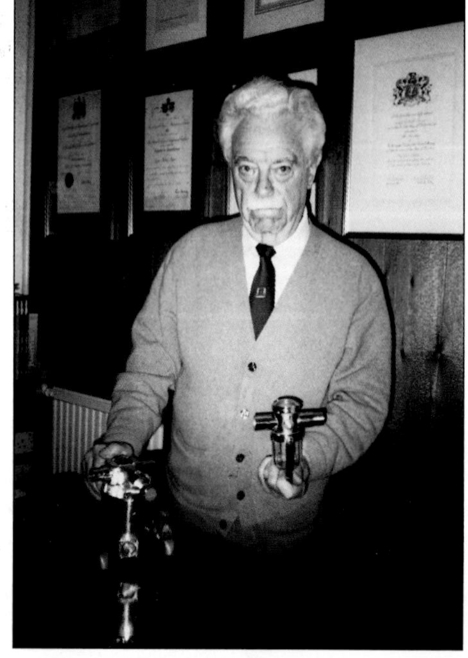

Professor J.P. Payne holding a Goldman vaporiser and with the Chlorotec vaporiser (on the table) he used until his retirement in 1987. (*Author's collection, photograph taken by kind permission of Professor J.P. Payne*)

under anaesthetic. These mildly stimulating tales often described otherwise modest patients uttering passionate endearments or even offering to embrace the virtuously embarrassed practitioner, whose spotless reputation was only maintained by the presence of respectable witnesses. In these stories it is almost always women who seem to be affected by inappropriate desires, and no mention is ever made of male patients uttering endearments to nurses.

Dudley Wilmot Buxton, an anaesthetist of considerable experience and influence, pointed out that all anaesthetics:

> . . . possess the power of exciting sexual emotions, and in many cases produce erotic hallucinations. It is undoubted that in certain persons sexual orgasm may occur during the induction of anaesthesia. Women, especially, when suffering from ovarian or uterine irritation, are prone to such hallucinations, and it is almost impossible to convince them after their recovery to consciousness that the subjective sexual sensation is not of objective existence.[3]

Where criminal charges were brought they usually amounted to little more than the patient's word against that of the doctor, and only rarely led to a conviction. In 1858 Montreal dentist John Webster was tried for the rape of a Mrs Nichols while she was under the influence of chloroform. She was clearly convinced that he had achieved his purpose, even though she had been menstruating at the time, but there was no physical evidence that a rape had taken place. Medical witnesses testified that chloroform sometimes made women use foul language, and a Mr Goodrich gave evidence that his wife had also accused Webster of rape after dental work, even though he (Goodrich) had been with her the whole time. All in all, it seemed that Webster was a true gentleman, and the only thing that could be said against him was that Mrs Nichols had been left unattended on a couch for an hour and a half after her tooth extraction. The judge summed up in Webster's favour. He said that rape had been ruled out, and they had only to decide if there had been an attempt. In view of the lack of evidence he advised that they should give Webster the benefit of the doubt. Quite what the jury was thinking of we shall never know, but they found Webster guilty of attempted rape and then made a recommendation for mercy. Juries have done stranger things – but not very often.[4]

Possibly the best-known doctor to find himself accused of rape under chloroform was Sir William Wilde, father of Oscar, and noted both as an ear and eye surgeon, and for his many extramarital affairs. In 1864 a sensational trial caused great excitement in Dublin. Mary Travers, a patient of Sir William, had first consulted him in 1854 when she was eighteen. She claimed that she had been violated in 1862, after being given chloroform in his study. Despite this, she had continued to visit him, and asked to borrow money. In 1864 Mary published her allegations in a pamphlet, and engaged newsboys to distribute copies. The Wildes chose not to prosecute Mary; instead, Lady Wilde wrote to Mary's father accusing her of disreputable conduct. Mary sued her for libel and the whole matter was debated in open court. When questioned about the incident, Mary no longer claimed that Sir William had used chloroform, saying that she had become unconscious when Sir William had placed his hand roughly between the ribbon of her bonnet and her neck. She explained that her pamphlet had said that he had used chloroform because she 'had to think of something treacherous' and had hit on chloroform as being better than the truth. This frank admission of lying should have settled the matter at once in Lady Wilde's favour, but instead the jury found for Miss Travers and awarded her damages of one farthing, while Sir William, since a husband was then liable for his wife's debts, found himself with a bill for £2,000 in legal costs.[5]

Despite the official view that accusations against doctors were either malicious or delusional, there remain some cases which suggest that not all medical men were paragons of virtue. In June 1870, Richard Thomas Freeman, a 33-year-old surgeon of Deptford, found himself on trial charged with the sexual assault of 24-year-old Lucy Ashby.[6] Miss Ashby, the daughter of a respectable local tradesman, had been in the company of a young man on Easter Monday. Accused by her mother of improper sexual conduct, and her virtue called into question, there was only one way of disproving the charges – an intimate examination by a doctor. Accompanied by her father, Miss Ashby went to Freeman's consulting rooms and requested an examination. Freeman agreed and her father waited outside for about half an hour. It does not seem to have struck him that this was an unusually long time. When he eventually went in to see his daughter, Freeman assured him that everything was satisfactory, but Lucy at once made a complaint. She said that when she had entered the room she had been asked to sit in a low chair, and Freeman had given her a bottle of something to smell. The fragrance of the liquid was like the taste of apples, and when she shook the bottle, some of it went over her chin and burnt her skin. She inhaled as she was told, and after a time became stupefied. When she opened her eyes she saw Freeman standing over her holding an instrument that he said he had been using on her. Her clothing was in disarray, and she was sure she had been assaulted. Freeman at once accused her of telling lies, but Lucy and her father went to another doctor who examined her. There must have been physical evidence of assault, for Freeman was arrested.

Freeman was in some difficulty. On his own statement in front of a witness it could be proved that Lucy had not been sexually active prior to the visit to his surgery, but almost immediately afterwards a second doctor had given evidence which had placed him in the dock. Surely the jury could not ignore this? The only defence that could be made was an attack on Lucy Ashby's mental state. At the trial it was claimed that she had a hysterical temperament and was subject to delusions, and also that the nature of the examination could have affected her brain. A shop boy was brought to say that chloroform had never been used at all, which if it were the case did not help Freeman, as it ruled out anaesthetic hallucination.

In the face of the medical evidence, the jury found the prisoner not guilty and the judge admonished him never to undertake such an examination again except in the presence of other persons. Which only goes to show that at the very least Richard Thomas Freeman was incapable of learning his lesson, for it so happened that he had been tried for a similar offence only three years previously.[7]

In 1867, Mary Ann Warren, a twenty-year-old servant, attended Freeman's surgery to have some teeth removed. She was asked to sit on a low chair, and something was administered to her in an inhaler. She awoke, half on and half off the chair, her skirts raised to her shoulders, with Dr Freeman taking criminal liberties which the newspapers declined to describe. She lost consciousness again, and when she came to, her clothes had been put back in order and her mouth was bleeding from the tooth extraction. Freeman then went out of the room and asked his servant to come in and look after the patient. Her mistress soon arrived to take her home, but Mary, who felt unwell, made no complaint at the time. On the following day, however, she told her mother what had happened and showed her the state of her underclothes. Mary went with her married sister to Guy's Hospital, where an examination showed that there were internal injuries of a recent date. The defence was that she was a 'corrupt perjurer', and that she had been intimate with another man and was trying to blame the doctor. The servant, who Mary had said was not in the room during the operation, gave evidence that she had been in the room the whole time. There were witnesses to state that Mary had been to the park with a young man, and this was enough for the jury to give Freeman the benefit of the doubt. Whatever the truth of these cases, Freeman must have learned to exercise caution with female patients. The 1881 census return shows him still practising medicine. He must have realised that a third trial might not go in his favour.

The statements of eminent medical men could carry a trial even when conviction seemed inevitable. In 1877 Dr Benjamin Ward Richardson gave evidence in the trial of a surgeon's assistant called George Howard who had been charged with rape by 23-year-old Mrs Fanny Child, who had gone to him for a tooth extraction.[8] Richardson had no personal knowledge of the case, but had been called as an expert witness.

Mrs Child had gone to the surgery with a female friend, a Miss Fellows, who had been absent from the room for fifteen minutes. When Miss Fellows returned, the door, which had been ajar when she left, was latched, and she had to ring for admission. Mrs Child, still under the influence of the chloroform, was unable to talk, but as soon as she could she told her husband John that Howard had 'done all that he could to me'. Howard denied the charges, suggesting not only that Mrs Child was delusional, but that she herself had admitted to him that she was not sure of what had happened. This last claim was certainly untrue, since on next being confronted by Mrs Child she at once declared, 'It's no use your saying anything – you did it.' On the following day John Child again asked Howard to his home to discuss the accusation. He demanded that Howard make a full apology to his wife and also acknowledge what he had done. Howard hesitated, and at last said he was willing to make an apology but not the acknowledgement. This wasn't good enough for Child, who continued to demand the acknowledgement. Eventually Howard gave him what he wanted, not once, but three times. It must have been with some relief that Howard left the house, under the impression that the matter was now closed. As he walked down the street he heard the footsteps of John Child behind him, and suddenly found himself being placed in the custody of a policeman who, by prior arrangement, had been lurking outside the door.

At Howard's trial, Dr Richardson told the jury that he had known people have delusions under chloroform and mentioned an instance at which he had been present. The surgery must have been somewhat crowded on that occasion, as apart from himself, the dentist and the patient, her father and mother and an assistant had all been in the room. The lady, said Richardson, had made a similar charge, which in view of the many witnesses could not have been true. The production of delusions, he added, was one of the earliest objections to the use of chloroform, but he failed to mention the howls of derision that had greeted this suggestion. Other medical witnesses appeared, agreeing with Richardson, one of whom observed that 'in the case of the fair sex the delusions sometimes assume quite a scandalous form'.[9]

Howard was acquitted, the judge commenting, 'No one could now doubt that the prosecutrix honestly believed that she had been assaulted in the manner she had related, and no one could now doubt that she was mistaken in that belief.'[10]

CHLOROFORM AND THE VICE TRADE

In July 1885 there were extraordinary scenes outside the offices of the *Pall Mall Gazette*. The popular newspaper was virtually in a state of siege, obliged to lock and barricade its doors against the excited surging crowds. The reason was a four-part article entitled 'The Maiden Tribute of Modern Babylon',[11] a crusading exposure of child prostitution in England, the first part appearing in the issue of 6 July. The article described in shocking detail how children as young as thirteen were snared into a life of vice, drugged and raped.

While many readers praised the boldness of the *Gazette* in exposing corruption, others regarded the articles as pornography. 'Anything more disgusting I never read.' said one correspondent who was anxious lest his daughters saw it; another thought such articles would only be enjoyed by persons of 'depraved appetites'.[12] Other newspapers also denounced the *Pall Mall Gazette*, such as the *Leeds Mercury*, which, while not denying the good motives of 'the men who have sown this mass of filth broadcast upon the streets of the metropolis', nevertheless felt that any good done was 'outweighed a thousandfold by the evil which is wrought by the wholesale revelation of indescribable vice'.[13] Many newsagents refused to stock the *Gazette*, which was why the offices were suddenly besieged, and copies were printed and reprinted until the presses ran out of paper.

The *Gazette*'s trump card was played in the issue of 6 July. This concluded with a section entitled 'A Child of Thirteen Bought for £5', which described how a drunken mother had eagerly sold her virgin daughter, named 'Lily', for that sum. No one could accuse the writer of believing unverifiable tales from dubious sources, for the purchaser was an agent of the *Pall Mall Gazette*, who had bought the child to save her from a life of shame.

The author of the article was William Thomas Stead, a crusading journalist of great energy and passion, editor of the *Pall Mall Gazette* since 1880. Born in 1849, the son of a Congregationalist minister, Stead was, on his own admission, 'mad about sex'. He was a friend of Havelock Ellis, who was to write *Studies in the Psychology of Sex*, and when the two men talked of an evening it appeared that they spoke of little else.[14]

Stead lived a strictly moral life, but was able to do so only by the exercise of self-control and diverting his energies into his work. 'The mastery of sexuality was a great problem with him. His repressed sexuality was, I consider, the motive force of many of his activities,' said Ellis.[15] Stead particularly attacked vice and prostitution, which he described as 'the ghastliest curse which haunts civilised society'.[16] Denying himself indulgence in sin, he was attacking the very thing that troubled him.

Stead's journalistic style was quite unlike the dry content of his rival newspapers. Eloquent and bold, full of fire and enthusiasm, he denounced social evils as if from a pulpit. He was only a part of the larger reform movement of the 1880s, which included such notables as Josephine Butler, leader of the Ladies National Association and W. Bramwell Booth, Chief of Staff of the Salvation Army. In 1885 the age of consent was only thirteen; a Bill was to be brought before parliament to raise the age to sixteen but it was unlikely that it would be passed. It seemed that Members of Parliament did not believe that teenage prostitution was a serious problem. Stead determined to arouse public concern by carrying out and publishing his own research, and over a period of six weeks interviewed brothel-keepers and prostitutes. He was told that young girls were acquired by enticing them under false pretences, when they were drugged either with snuff or laudanum in a drink of beer, or chloroform, and violated. One former brothel-keeper confidently assured him that in parts of London there were whole streets where drunken families were willing to sell their virgin daughters. There was only one way to prove that the vile trade existed, and that was to actually purchase a virgin, but when Stead asked his contact to deliver two girls to him, the man hesitated, and eventually offered two girls who were the daughters of brothel-keepers. Obviously it wasn't as simple as he had claimed.

Stead decided to engage the assistance of a Mrs Rebecca Jarrett, a lady who had once been a prostitute and kept a 'gay house', as brothels were then known, but now in her late thirties and lame she had rejected her old associates and was working with the Salvation Army to rescue girls from a life of vice. He had known her only a week, but she came with a testimonial from Josephine Butler herself, and Stead trusted her absolutely. Jarrett was given the task of acquiring a thirteen-year-old virgin, to demonstrate the ease with which a girl could be procured and placed in moral danger. It was essential that the girl should not be harmed or frightened, and that she should be led to believe that she was to be employed as a domestic servant. Stead was aware that he might be putting himself in danger of prosecution, and after taking legal advice was confident that as long as he had no criminal intent, he would be safe, and so set in train the events that would eventually land him and several others, including two well-meaning Salvation Army officers, in the dock of the Old Bailey.

Jarrett was unhappy about this task, not being especially willing to visit her old haunts. She also knew it would be difficult, as she had abandoned the life more than six months ago. An active procuress usually had a number of girls in training, but Jarrett had to start from nothing. Booth and Butler urged her to help, and Stead insisted – not only did he want it done, it had to be done soon, because of the impending Bill.

It took several days for Jarrett to return with a girl. Her initial attempts were unsuccessful, and on 2 June she eventually arrived on the doorstep of an old friend, Nancy Broughton, with whom she had once worked in a hotel laundry. Jarrett asked Nancy to put the word around that she was looking for a girl of about thirteen for a domestic place. Girls were brought to her, but she rejected them as too old. Then Eliza Armstrong, the thirteen-year-old daughter of a chimney-sweep, heard about the search, and as she was looking for work, brought her mother to see Jarrett about the position. Jarrett claimed that she needed a servant as she had a large house in Wimbledon, but Mrs Armstrong declared that this was too far away and wouldn't let Eliza go. On the following day, Jarrett returned. It was Derby Day, a fact which later helped to fix the date in people's memories. In the interval, Eliza had pestered her mother to let her take the position. Mrs Armstrong eventually relented and when Jarrett arrived went to see her.

This is the point where the stories diverge. According to Mrs Armstrong, she was always under the impression that Eliza was going into domestic service, and the only money she received was when Mrs Jarrett gave her a shilling to buy something for her baby. She had only agreed to let her daughter go because Nancy Broughton had vouched for her friend's character. Jarrett, on the other hand, said that when Eliza was not present, she had made it plain to the mother that the girl was going to an immoral life, and gave £1 to Mrs Armstrong for the girl and £4 to Nancy as a procuress. Nancy Broughton's version of the conversation entirely supported Mrs Armstrong.

Jarrett bought some new clothes for Eliza, and took her away. When Charles Armstrong arrived home and found Eliza had gone he expressed his feelings in his usual fashion by hitting his wife.

A great deal of what we know about what followed comes from the evidence of young Eliza. Armed with no more than the most basic education, her composure, resilience, intelligence and keen observation were to be vital factors in the downfall of William Stead.

It was an essential part of Stead's scheme that he should be able to show that a young virgin could be placed in moral danger, so he needed proof that little Eliza was indeed pure. This task he entrusted to Jarrett, together with Sampson Jacques, a Greek war correspondent who had been introduced to Stead because of their mutual interest in exposing the vice trade. In Jacques's investigations he had become acquainted with Mme Louise

Mourey, an elderly French lady who called herself a midwife, but had once been a procuress and abortionist, and boasted of her proficiency in certifying virgins. Stead and Jacques wanted to prove to society that such a creature existed; therefore it was to this lady that the child was taken for certification of her purity. Eliza was briefly left alone with Mme Mourey who, without any warning of what was to happen, and much to the child's disgust, carried out the examination. For this service she charged 20 shillings, and, before they left, she sold Jacques a small bottle of chloroform, about a shilling's worth, saying that her clients always found it most effective. For this, she demanded 30 shillings. Eliza was then removed in a cab to a house in Poland Street, which she was told was a hotel, but was in fact a brothel.

The next step of the plan was to show that it was possible for a man to enter the girl's bedroom, and Stead (for he was to be the man) was anxious that Eliza was not to be alarmed. Having committed abduction and indecent assault, the 'secret commission', as Stead called them, added an attempt to administer a noxious substance to the catalogue of their crimes. Eliza was persuaded to go to bed, and curtains were drawn around her. Jarrett lay down beside her fully dressed, sprinkled some chloroform on a handkerchief, and held it to the girl's nose. Eliza pushed it away, but Jarrett tried again, saying it was scent, and asking Eliza to take a good sniff. Eliza didn't like the smell and threw the handkerchief away. Stead, who had been hovering outside waiting for his cue, assumed that Eliza was asleep, and walked in. She at once sat up and screamed: 'There's a man in the room!'

Stead darted out again, and Jarrett lifted the curtain and said: 'There's no man there.'

'Because he's gone out,' said Eliza, firmly.[17]

By now Stead must have concluded he had made his point and Eliza was quickly whisked away. In his defence speech before the magistrate, Stead gave the following description of that night's events:

> [Mrs Jarrett] dressed her and took her to a respectable house, where she passed the night. That was all that passed in that brothel. Eliza Armstrong passed out as pure as she entered it, not exactly knowing whether 'the man' had really been in the room or whether it was a mere vision of the night. No hand

> was laid upon her to do her harm. Had she been my own daughter I could not have been more careful to shield her from the very suspicion of evil.[18]

This was true as far as it went, but Stead had very carefully made an important omission. The full details of what happened to Eliza later that night did not emerge for several months, and were something that Stead was clearly anxious to conceal.

The following day she was placed in the care of the Salvation Army, whose officers were informed that her drunken mother had sold her into prostitution and she was in need of protection. Bramwell Booth arranged for a Mrs Combe, a wealthy Swiss lady engaged in charity work, to accompany Eliza to France where she was given employment. On 10 June Jarrett deflected enquiry by sending a postcard to Nancy Broughton to say that Eliza was all right.

In 'The Maiden Tribute', Stead wrote, 'I can personally vouch for the absolute accuracy of every fact in the narrative'[19] but, dangerously, he was vouching for events at which he had not been present. Jarrett had given Stead a detailed account of how Eliza had been procured, but there was no documentary evidence, and Stead, who prided himself on an excellent memory, took no notes of the conversation. It was another four weeks before he wrote his article.

In his narrative, Jarrett's old friend Nancy Broughton becomes a brothel-keeper, Mrs Armstrong is 'poor, dissolute, and indifferent to everything but drink'[20] and, with full understanding of the nature of the transaction, offers her own daughter for a life of prostitution, for the sum of £3, with £2 to follow when virginity was certified. Charles Armstrong, who was not even present during the negotiations, was represented as knowing all about them, but drunk and indifferent. All these people had good grounds to take action for libel, and substantial out of court settlements were to follow.

Alarmingly, Stead reported of Jarrett that 'unaccustomed to anything but drugging by the administration of sleeping potions, she would infallibly have poisoned the child had she not discovered by experiment that the liquid burned the mouth when an attempt was made to swallow it'.[21] Nevertheless he goes on to state that Jarrett, who minutes earlier was dangerously ignorant of the use of chloroform, successfully put

Eliza to sleep with it: 'She was rather restless, but under the influence of chloroform she soon went over.'[22] By now, Stead's narrative has more holes in it than a Skinner mask, for having claimed that Eliza was asleep, he could not omit the dramatic scene where she sensed that there was a man in her room and cried out piteously for help.

Stead's article achieved everything he could have hoped. It aroused enormous public indignation about the trade in young girls. Protest meetings were held all over the country, and there was a mass demonstration in Hyde Park. On 14 August 1885 the previously neglected Bill to raise the age of consent passed into law by a huge majority.

Stead, very much the hero of the hour, addressed a public meeting on 21 August, saying, 'We took the child from a place steeped in vice, from a mother who has admitted that she was going to a brothel,'[23] thus adding slander to the growing list of his offences. It was the first public statement in which it was admitted that 'Lily' was indeed Eliza, and Stead was happy to take full responsibility for everything that had occurred. A few days later, Stead, Jarrett, Jacques, Mme Mourey, Bramwell Booth and Mrs Combe were all under arrest.

When Mrs Armstrong had seen the *Pall Mall Gazette* in July, she became afraid that the child reported as having been sold on Derby Day was her daughter. Even her neighbours saw the coincidence and gave her a hard time. If she had indeed been an alcoholic who had callously sold her child into prostitution, it would have been easy for her to deny that 'Lily' was Eliza. Instead, Mrs Armstrong had a ferocious row with Nancy Broughton, and reported her daughter missing. Her plight was soon publicised by *Lloyd's Newspaper*, which scented scandal. Jarrett had sent another postcard which stated that Eliza was doing well, and it was her notes that formed the first clues in a trail that led the police investigators to the Salvation Army. Eliza was traced to France, and when Stead found that Mrs Armstrong wanted her back, the girl was brought home and, on 24 August, reunited with her mother.

Stead was still maintaining that Eliza has been successfully chloroformed by Jarrett, for he wrote in the *Pall Mall Gazette*, 'She smelt the chloroform bottle and dozed off into a gentle slumber, from which she unfortunately woke with a start when I entered the room.'[24]

On 2 September, at Bow Street magistrates court, Jarrett was formally charged with abduction, indecent assault and 'administering and causing to be administered to, and taken by, Eliza Armstrong, a certain noxious thing with intent to injure, aggrieve, and annoy her'[25] and conspiring with William Thomas Stead and others to commit these offences.

By now, the *Pall Mall Gazette*'s rival newspapers had started to turn public opinion against Stead, and people were beginning to wonder if the whole affair had been a fraud from the start. Crowds estimated at 2,000 in number collected around the Old Bailey to jeer at the defendants, and when Mrs Armstrong gave evidence, alternately weeping and angry, she shook her fist at Jarrett, saying she would 'let her have it', an action that brought a burst of applause in court.[26]

Stead was initially confident that he would be vindicated. When he had written 'The Maiden Tribute', the Armstrongs and Nancy Broughton were shadowy figures, caricatures sketched partly from Jarrett's description and partly from his own imagination. He now had to face and understand them as human beings. The defence sought to establish the character of the daily life of the neighbourhood and elicited from the Armstrongs that they had been known to drink and to swear and that Armstrong hit his wife, yet it was obvious that neither of them was indifferent to the fate of their daughter. The first major blow to Stead's confidence must have come with the evidence of the policeman, Inspector Borner, who described how Mrs Armstrong had been distressed and frantic about the fate of her child.

As the hearing drew to a close Stead had accepted that some at least of the things he had written in 'The Maiden Tribute' were untrue. He now described how a decidedly conscious Eliza had thrown away the chloroformed handkerchief, adding, with a dismissive flourish, 'that, according to the story of the prosecution, is the administering of a drug which figures so prominently in the summons'[27], ignoring the fact that the accusation originated from his own personally vouched-for account. Stead actually had the very bottle on his person, which he handed to the surprised prosecuting counsel. This slightly flippant dismissal of the chloroforming charge reads very uncomfortably in the light of later revelations. The truth would explode upon Stead and others at the trial.

His trust in Jarrett had obviously received a knock for he added, 'Whether I was right or wrong in believing the report which Rebecca Jarrett brought me concerning the negotiations by which the child came into her possession is a point on which opinions may differ. There can, however be no question as to the sincerity with which I accepted the report of my agent.'[28]

The defendants were sent for trial, although Bramwell Booth and Mrs Combe were, to what must have been their immense relief, not asked to answer charges of indecent assault, and the charge of administering a noxious substance was not pursued at all.

The trial opened on 23 October, with Stead defending himself, and from his point of view things went from bad to worse. He admitted that the section in 'The Maiden Tribute' about a child purchased for £5 referred to Eliza, and that for the truth of the story he had relied entirely on the verbal statement of Rebecca Jarrett. His accusation that Nancy Broughton was a procuress and her house a brothel was now shown to be quite untrue, as Jarrett, saying 'I think Mr Stead has made some slight mistakes in the article',[29] admitted that she had never known her friend do anything improper, and denied having told Stead many of the details he had published. She even expressed her doubts that 'Lily' was actually Eliza, and suggested that she might be another child entirely.

By contrast with the plain-speaking Armstrongs and Nancy Broughton, Jarrett made a poor impression. Asked about where she had kept 'improper houses' she first gave three addresses which when checked were found to be false. Questioned again, she accused counsel of forcing her to lie, and then refused point blank to answer any further questions about her past life.

Stead later admitted, 'I am now somewhat shaken in Jarrett, I have not the implicit trust in her memory that I had. Her memory seems defective, I think she intended to tell the truth.'[30]

He continued to maintain that his story was substantially true, that Mrs Armstrong had agreed for Eliza to be taken away in full knowledge of what was intended, but when Mr Justice Lopes ruled that 'parental consent' meant the father's consent the case was effectively lost even if it had not been so before. The only evidence that the child had been sold into prostitution was that of Jarrett, who had been shown to be a liar.

On 27 October the gynaecologist Dr Heywood Smith, who had been issued with a subpoena, took the stand and revealed just what had happened after Eliza had been removed from the brothel.[31] Stead had contacted him about the project as long ago as the previous May. Knowing that he might be accused of having violated the girl, Stead had asked Smith to certify the girl's virginity as soon as she left the brothel. Because Eliza had been alarmed and removed rather earlier than planned, this had had to be organised very quickly. The house she had been taken to was a nursing home. The nurse in charge, a Miss Hutchinson, had been roused out of bed by the night bell. She prepared beds for Eliza and Jarrett, and was told to expect the arrival of a doctor. While Eliza and Jarrett slept, Miss Hutchinson was obliged to sit up until Smith's arrival at 3 a.m. when she conducted him to the bedroom. Jarrett was awoken to act as a witness, and Smith gave Hutchinson some chloroform and a handkerchief and asked her to chloroform Eliza without waking her up. He then left the room. The nurse did as she was told, although it later transpired when she gave evidence that she had never given chloroform before, only seen it done. Smith returned and took over the handkerchief, and Hutchinson, after supplying him with a pot of Vaseline, retired from the room.[32] He then carried out an intimate examination of the unconscious girl. It only remained for him to write out a certificate of virginity, which he sent to Bramwell Booth, and a bill for 3 guineas, which was later paid by Stead. It would not have been surprising if the jury had wondered whether Smith and possibly also Hutchinson should have been in the dock beside Mme Mourey.

Stead declined to question both these witnesses, but when he next addressed the jury realised that some explanation was required, and said he had asked for the examination to protect the reputation of himself and Mr Booth. 'The examination inflicted no pain, nor did one foul thought sully the mind of Eliza Armstrong,' claimed Stead.[33] An interesting comment in the light of Dr Richardson's opinions – apparently chloroform could both stimulate sexual feelings in women and prevent them as gentlemen found it convenient!

Unsurprisingly, the verdict of the jury was that Eliza had been taken away without her father's consent, and they also found that her mother had not sold her into prostitution. Mr Justice Lopes, while recognising Stead's altruistic motives, had to take into account the suffering that had been inflicted on a respectable family. The end, he believed, did not sanctify the means, and in his opinion 'The Maiden Tribute' was a series of 'disgusting and filthy articles – articles so filthy and so disgusting that one cannot help fearing that they may have suggested to innocent women and children the existence of vice and wickedness which had never occurred to their minds before'.[34]

He also censured Dr Smith, whom he believed had brought discredit to his profession, although he absolved Miss Hutchinson of any blame. Stead was imprisoned for three months. Jarrett, said Lopes, had misled her employer but he felt that she had done so after having taken on the task under some pressure. She was imprisoned for six months. Jacques was found not guilty of the abduction but guilty of indecent assault and was imprisoned for a month. For Louise Mourey, Lopes saved his harshest words and imprisoned her for six months with hard labour. She died in prison the following January, aged seventy-four. Bramwell Booth and Mrs Combe were acquitted of all charges.

The *Lancet*, which usually defended its own, was appalled that a child had been placed at risk solely to preserve the reputation of Mr Stead, and roundly condemned Dr Smith for actions tantamount to indecent assault.[35] Smith unwisely argued that Professor Simpson had once suggested chloroform could be given for intimate examinations to spare the feelings of the patient.[36] The *Lancet* pointed out very bluntly that Eliza had not been Dr Smith's patient, he had not sought the permission of her parents, and the examination had not been for any medical purpose.[37] Smith was later obliged to resign as secretary of the British Gynaecological Society, and was dismissed from his post at the British Lying-in Hospital, the entire committee having threatened to resign as a body if he was permitted to remain.[38] The final penalty was an official reprimand by the Royal College of Physicians, from which he was very fortunate not to be ejected.[39] This sorry episode is sanitised in a single line in Stead's official biography – 'she was again examined, this time by a well-known physician Dr Heywood Smith, who certified that she had suffered no injury of any kind'.[40]

Stead, whatever his private opinion of Jarrett, later wrote, 'That Rebecca Jarrett, with her muddled brain and defective memory, had misled me, intentionally or otherwise, was indubitable after the conflict of our evidence.'[41] He never seems to have understood that she might have been forced into a deception by his insistence on her carrying out a difficult and sensitive task in an impossibly short time. He was released from prison in January 1886, but his reputation had suffered, and the *Pall Mall Gazette* was never quite what it had once been. The circulation fell, and in 1890 Stead resigned and became the editor of the *Review of Reviews*. Years later Eliza wrote to him saying she was married to a good man and had six children. Stead remained a campaigning journalist and pioneer of reform to the end of his life. He travelled widely, and in April 1912 set out for America on the *Titanic*. As the stricken ship sank, he helped women and children into the lifeboats but made no attempt to save himself.

When Rebecca Jarrett was released from prison, she was welcomed back to service with the Salvation Army, and after a long and honourable career she died in 1928, aged eighty-one.

TEN

The Joy of Ether

Is it not time, Sir, that the profession should determine to discountenance and discontinue the use of chloroform and other dangerous anaesthetics and have recourse alone to the administration of ether in operations of any duration?

Letter from George Pollock to the Lancet, *2 December 1874*[1]

When Dr Benjamin Joy Jeffries arrived in England in August 1872 he was a man with a mission. Born in Boston, he had studied at Harvard and practised as an ophthalmic surgeon at the Massachusetts Eye and Ear Infirmary. Joy Jeffries, as he was usually known, was well aware of the frequency of chloroform deaths in Europe, and believed that the only reason English and continental surgeons persisted in its use was their unfamiliarity with ether. Although he was in London to attend an international conference of ophthalmologists, he had another, much bolder purpose, to single-handedly bring about the abandonment of chloroform as an anaesthetic. He very nearly succeeded.

In the UK, surgeons had largely given up the search for the perfect anaesthetic and were concentrating their efforts on improved means of resuscitation. Galvanism (electric current) had its adherents, as did artificial respiration, although Dr Richardson believed that rough handling could paralyse the heart, and preferred inflating the lungs, either by mouth, or with a little bellows of his own devising (price 10 shillings). Another widely used method was inverting the patient to allow blood to flow to the head. Brandy, wine, ice or the surgeon's thumb were sometimes inserted into the patient's rectum, and those well-known 'stimulants' brandy and ether were also given by injection. Whatever the preference, reports of chloroform deaths show that when faced with a lifeless patient, frantic doctors tried every method at their disposal.

Time had done nothing to erase the London/Edinburgh divide. There was suspicion in England that Scottish doctors were being less than open about the numbers of chloroform deaths, and in 1871 the *British Medical Journal* openly challenged Dr Gillespie of the Edinburgh Royal Infirmary, who had claimed that a recent death was the first in his practice since the introduction of chloroform.[2] Gillespie was forced to admit that he had had another in his private practice, and did not respond to the assertion that there had been at least four or five other deaths in the Infirmary. The *British Medical Journal*, stating that chloroform had proved to be about six or seven times as dangerous as it was originally hoped to be, suggested that it should no longer be used in dentistry, while for surgery it was time to re-examine the use of ether.[3] This was the first shot in what was to become an extended campaign by that journal for the reintroduction of ether, but the moment was not right, and few gave it any consideration.

Alternatives had been tried and found wanting. Mixtures of chloroform and ether were occasionally used but were thought to be unreliable, because it was impossible to know exactly what the patient was inhaling. A few British surgeons used ether, but most of those who tried it were unhappy both with the time it took and the depth of anaesthesia, and went back to using chloroform.

In the United States, ether, applied using a sponge in a cone of towelling or paper to protect the patient's face, had long been considered safe and simple. Such was the confidence in the process that it was not thought to require a specialist, and was often entrusted to a nurse or a medical student. The capital city of ether was undoubtedly Boston, where in 1870 an anonymous contributor to the *Boston Medical and Surgical Journal* headed his article 'Homicides by Chloroform'[4] commenting, 'A good trial for manslaughter by a New England jury would bring British doctors to a quickened sense of responsibility . . .'.

In the chloroform-using countries of the world, years of quibbling over the patient's posture, the ambient temperature, and the pre-operative breakfast had done nothing to stop the deaths. For many years the actual death rate due to chloroform was a matter of guesswork and conjecture, but in 1870 Benjamin

Ward Richardson, with details of some 80,000 operations, came up with the alarming statistic of one death per 2,500 uses.[5]

Hope was fading that a better and more accurate inhaler would appear and solve the problem, and in 1873 the *Lancet* had a shocking confession to make.[6] For the last sixteen years, that august journal had been warning surgeons against the dangers of administering chloroform on a handkerchief, sponge or lint, insisting that the best guarantee of safety was to use an inhaler. As death followed death, so editorials were written roundly chastising the readership for not following advice that must surely reduce the mortality rate. It was now felt necessary to admit that the method of administration made little or no difference. In this, the editor was almost certainly echoing the conclusion that his readers had already reached.

Matters may have been brought to a head by a recent death during the use of Clover's apparatus.[7] It was later admitted that the bellows used to fill the bag had been stiff, and only gave 8,400 cubic inches of air and not 11,000. The intended proportion of chloroform vapour to air had been 2.8 per cent but the patient had actually received 3.67 per cent. Since this was still less than Snow's recommended maximum, this highly unsatisfactory explanation must have had anxious surgeons reaching thankfully for their Skinner masks.

The main difficulty with Clover's apparatus was its size and expense. While suited to a hospital environment, a doctor could hardly fold it into his hat for transport. Clover, the skilful and highly respected leader of anaesthesia in London, was convinced that his carefully measured percentages were the only way of ensuring safety. In Scotland, however, his opinions were to provoke the wrath of one of the great men of medicine, Sir Joseph (later Baron) Lister, whose introduction of the antiseptic system in surgery put an end at last to the belief in laudable pus. Lister had his own very firm ideas on how to administer chloroform, which matched those of his late father-in-law Dr Syme, and the stage was set for open conflict.

Lister's writing on anaesthesia is confident and bombastic, not so much bordering on arrogance but marching through with bagpipes skirling. His mode of administration was simplicity itself: 'A common towel being arranged so as to form a square cloth of six folds, enough chloroform is poured upon it to moisten a surface in the middle about as large as the palm of the hand, the precise quantity used being a matter of no consequence whatever.'[8] Despite this cavalier attitude he believed that 'Death from chloroform is *almost invariably* due to faulty administration.'[9]

He also claimed that no deaths had occurred in the Edinburgh and Glasgow infirmaries,[10] which the *British Medical Journal* pointed out was untrue.[11] To Lister, it was all very simple. The only cause of death was paralysis of the respiration and the only remedy was pulling the tongue forward with a pair of artery forceps, the resultant hole in the patient's tongue being a trivial matter in view of the emergency. To be fair, Lister had personally saved lives by this method, but he was so assured of his rightness that he dismissed as illusory the overwhelming evidence of sudden death by cardiac arrest, saying:

> The evidence of bystanders is apt to be conflicting with regard to the precise succession of highly important events that are crowded together in the brief period of excitement immediately preceding death, and there is also a strong tendency that exists in the mind of anyone in whose hands such a case has occurred, to twist the evidence, unconsciously to himself, in favour of inevitable syncope, rather than preventable asphyxia.[12]

In other words, Lister believed that doctors who had failed to treat asphyxia were deluding themselves into believing that the actual cause of death was something else which they could do nothing about. He did have a point. Ordinary practitioners who did not enjoy Lister's profound self-belief approached the process of anaesthesia with great anxiety. They did their best, they followed all the advice in the journals, but sometimes it just wasn't enough, and then they found themselves accused of professional negligence. Many still clung to the 'fatty heart' theory, and where that could not be found, fell back on that catch-all explanation of the Victorian doctor for every result he could not explain – an idiosyncrasy of the patient impossible to detect in life.

Lister was able to point to the death-free record both of himself and his illustrious father-in-law. He did not mention that Syme had had a few narrow escapes, but then he would not have seen them as such. In more than one of Syme's operations there had been a flutter or even a momentary cessation of the patient's pulse when the first incision was made.[13]

Clover, who believed that chloroform stopped the pulse before respiration, disagreed entirely with Lister's use of towel and forceps. He said that he had never needed to draw the tongue forward, and if Lister did then his method of giving chloroform wasn't the best one. When Clover thought the airway was being blocked by the tongue, he lifted the patient's chin, an action which remains a standard procedure to this day.[14] Lister called this 'about as pernicious a piece of advice as can well be given'.[15]

Anxious to discover how the obstruction occurred, Lister had chloroformed a sheep in a Glasgow slaughterhouse and cut its throat to enable him to look at the organs in action. (Matters were brought to an early close by the arrival of an official who threatened to have him up before the Provost and magistrates for such cruelty to animals.)[16] This, and observing the results of pulling his own tongue convinced him that his method was valid. Stung by the suggestion that overdoses occurred when chloroform was applied on a towel, Lister conducted a series of experiments to measure the percentage of vapour inhaled by a patient from the underside of a cloth, and concluded that it was below 4.5 per cent.[17] Allowing for the fact that not all was inhaled, he claimed that the patient was actually receiving as little or possibly even less than the amounts provided by Clover's apparatus. So far from being the 'harmless luxury' he had once thought it, he now suggested it might be responsible for overdose.[18]

Clover naturally took serious issue with this,[19] and London doctors sided with him, many openly attacking Lister's teachings as dangerous. Thomas Jones commented that since his first article was written, Lister had met with two or three cases which had almost proved fatal, and 'this seems to have shaken his mind'.[20]

Lister had been forced to admit that 'here and there an individual may be found so constituted that without any undue proportion of the narcotic vapour to the air inhaled, the cardiac ganglia may fail before the respiration is interfered with'.[21] In other words – idiosyncrasy. While all this was happening, however, a revolution was taking place.

On 24 October 1871, at a meeting of the Royal Medical and Chirurgical Society, J. Warrington Haward of St George's Hospital had delivered a paper on that neglected (in the UK) anaesthetic, ether, contending that it was safer than chloroform as it didn't paralyse the heart.[22] Although he spoke from personal experience, he met with a decidedly lukewarm reception from his fellow members, whose attitudes one assumes were typical of the time. One said he had tried ether and given it up, as it had made the patient excited and caused congestion of the chest. Others felt that the smell was an inconvenience. None was convinced that it was safer than chloroform, having no data on that subject. When that data was finally to arrive it was to take everyone by surprise.

Into this fertile bed breezed Joy Jeffries, who read a conference paper entitled 'Ether in Ophthalmic Surgery', emphasising that ether was as effectual as chloroform, as simple to use if one knew the right way, and, above all, risk-free. His advice, however, was somewhat alarming:

> When the patient, whether old or young, struggles, and asks for a respite and fresh air, do not yield. Hold them down by main force if necessary, and at any rate, keep the sponge tight over the mouth and nose till they finally take long breaths and go off into ether-sleep . . . my personal experience tells me that those who use chloroform have somehow a sort of dread of ether, as if it was to be suddenly fatal, and hence fail to give a patient enough to intoxicate him quickly.[23]

True, there had been deaths in the USA thought to be due to ether, but Jeffries confidently assured his audience that all had been investigated and all could be explained as due to something else. Ether, he declared, was absolutely safe.

The English ophthalmic surgeon Robert Brudenell Carter made a polite response. He felt that ether did not produce sufficient muscular relaxation. Having tried it, he had laid it aside returning to 'our old and trusted friend chloroform'. Nevertheless, Carter made a very important invitation. He asked Jeffries to come to St George's Hospital and demonstrate the use of ether, so they could see if their dissatisfaction was due to a fault in their administration. This very generous and humble request was exactly the chance Jeffries had hoped for, and during the remainder of his stay he was to give seventeen demonstrations in London hospitals. Using a towel rolled into a cone with a sponge at its apex, he decided to emphasise his total confidence in ether by pouring it on more lavishly than usual, with no attempt at measuring quantities. Unable to resist a look at the audience reaction he was gratified and not a little amused at the sea of shocked expressions.

After the demonstrations, which were entirely successful, he was bombarded with questions, one of which related to the relative expense of ether and chloroform. Jeffries believed that they were not much different, and was too polite to observe that any gentleman who had had a fatal case from chloroform would gladly deduct the difference in price from his own fee to avoid another. Jeffries had a question of his own to ask – what was the object of measuring the chloroform? He was told, with a smile, 'For the benefit of the coroner's jury.' He also revealed to his astonished audience that he was not a specialist etherist, but a surgeon. In America, he said, there was no need for a specialist as ether was so safe that it could be given by the surgeon himself, an assistant, or even a student.[24]

By the time Joy Jeffries returned to the USA, the movement he had started was in full swing. Surgeons who had distrusted chloroform, but been resigned to the fact that there was no good alternative, at once abandoned its use, and many more determined to at least give ether a trial. A few decided to use ether for the dangerous induction stage, but continue with chloroform, and since ether was thought to be a stimulant to the heart's action, kept some by to restore the patient if the pulse seemed to be failing. Others liked to start with a few whiffs of chloroform, and then continue with ether. There were enough examples of deaths under ether to cast doubt on Jeffries's claim that it was entirely safe, but Dr John Morgan, of St George's Hospital, combined American and British statistics and showed that chloroform deaths were 1 in 2,873 while those from ether were 1 in 23,204.[25]

In November 1872 the *British Medical Journal* observed 'Three weeks ago the administration of ether was a rare exception; we have reason to believe that it is already becoming the rule.'[26] The journals suddenly began to feature designs for new ether inhalers.

Not everyone embraced ether. Chloroform had the boon of ease and familiarity and it was possible for those who did not trust statistics to simply ignore them. There were, and would remain, surgeons who were passionate in their adherence to chloroform; thus a speaker at the Royal Medical Institution of Liverpool openly criticised the *British Medical Journal* for its 'unjustified crusade' against chloroform.[27] The *Lancet* was desperately out of touch. Its report on anaesthesia in November 1872 was dismissive of Dr Joy Jeffries, whom it called the 'apostle of the practice of employing ether', writing that he had said nothing which older experienced doctors had not heard many times before, and had mainly converted the young, to whom it was 'to some extent a novelty, and so it attracted'.[28] It followed this comment, somewhat pointedly, with an account of a death under ether, and then largely ignored the subject during the following year.

The sudden 'ether frenzy', as it was dubbed, caused a number of people to take a step back and wonder just why at the end of 1847 there had been a wholesale abandonment of ether for chloroform. Some were in no doubt about the identity of the villains of the piece. Dr Augustin Pritchard of Bristol named Professor James Miller, who had died in 1863, saying 'he helped to make the members of our profession blind to the risk of the agent'.[29] In 1879 a letter to the *British Medical Journal* expressed what many must have been thinking. 'It is by no means certain that the vulgarisation of chloroform by the energy of Simpson was not a disadvantage to humanity.'[30]

Matters were not moving fast enough for George Pollock, who decided to bring the matter into public debate by writing to *The Times*. Convinced that ether was completely safe, he was obviously frustrated by the failure of other surgeons to see his point of view. 'I ought perhaps to apologise for intruding a professional question on a non-professional journal,' he wrote, 'but one must employ a big hammer to drive a large nail though a thick piece of wood. We have some very thick pieces of wood to deal with.'[31]

In March 1875 Dr Fifield of Boston demonstrated the use of ether in Liverpool, which prompted Thomas Skinner to argue that Fifield as a Bostonian was prejudiced in favour of ether. In his own mind, of course, Skinner, as an ex-student of Simpson, was not prejudiced at all, he was simply right. Skinner was a great believer in the heroic administration of chloroform, pushing it into the patient as fast as he could take it, though he admitted that greater care was needed with 'delicate children and females of the middle and upper classes'.[32]

He had visited Boston in 1873 where a Dr Sinclair had told him that public opinion there was very much against chloroform, and he never used it, since if a patient of his died under its influence he was sure he would be tried for manslaughter.[33]

Angry at Fifield's denouncement of 'the greatest boon that

mankind ever received', Skinner called Boston 'the very hotbed of anti-chloroformism', and accused Fifield of being 'surcharged with purblind American prejudice, founded on fear, patriotism and ignorance.'[34]

He did, however, have a practical suggestion. Believing that chloroform deaths were entirely due to incompetence, he recommended that a committee be formed to agree upon a universal system of administration.

In August that year, at the Annual General Meeting of the British Medical Association, it was agreed that a committee should be appointed to enquire into and report upon the use of anaesthetics.[35] There were seven Scottish members, including Professor Lister, four English, including Clover, and two Irish. This committee was not able to meet for another two years, when it was pointed out that as the members came from London, Dublin, Edinburgh and Aberdeen, it was impossible for them to do what was required of them. This was presumably a reference to the geographical difficulty, though it is hard to see how a chloroform committee which included both Lister and Clover could ever agree on anything. As a result of this, a sub-committee was formed consisting entirely of Glasgow men, their remit being to report on the dangers of chloroform and find some safer anaesthetic. It was not to report for another three years.

By the end of 1875, it appeared that the dominance of chloroform in London, at least, was over.[36] The majority of hospitals were now using ether or a combination of nitrous oxide and ether as their anaesthetics of choice. A few hospitals such as Guy's still continued to use chloroform for most operations. Chloroform still remained dominant in Scotland for very many more years, and on the continent of Europe, which did not have its Joy Jeffries, the ether revolution never happened.

Even in hospitals where ether was normally the first choice, chloroform was still preferred for natural labour, and for the elderly and very young where the bronchial irritation caused by ether was a serious drawback. Ether's tendency to cause agitation had recognised dangers. A Dr McGill reported in 1873 that an elderly man who had been operated on under ether for a hernia, was briefly left alone to recover. On returning, the surgeon found that the patient had torn off his dressings and pulled two or three yards of intestine out of the wound, which were found lying in a glistening heap on the table beside him.

The complication proved fatal.[37] Chloroform was therefore used for operations where it was important to avoid movement, such as the setting of fractures.

Clover's inhaler was still in use, as were modified versions of Snow's, but there was a new kind of inhaler on the scene. Devised by F.E. Junker of the University of Vienna and the Royal Free Hospital, London, it soon became the most widely used apparatus for the administration of chloroform.[38] A small hand-held balloon pumped air through a rubber tube into a flask of anaesthetic, which was small enough to be hooked on to the administrator's lapel. The air bubbled through the liquid, and, laden with vapour, passed through a second rubber tube to a face-mask. Like Clover's apparatus it ensured that the chloroform did not evaporate directly over the mouth and nose of the patient, but it also had the enormous appeal of easy portability. There were complaints that the balloon and the mask required both the administrator's hands, thus apparently making it impossible for him to feel the pulse; however Junker declared that he could manage all three tasks with one hand. This feat of dexterity involved holding the mask while pressing the balloon against it with four fingers while feeling the facial artery with the fifth.[39] There were two serious drawbacks to Junker's inhaler. The two rubber tubes were so similar that it was quite possible to attach them the wrong way round, which resulted in liquid chloroform being pumped into the face-mask, and sometimes, into the patient. A similar accident could occur if the bottle tilted. There were several fatalities, since the surgeon was unlikely to be aware that anything was wrong until he saw liquid squirting out of the patient's mouth or surgical incision. Many modifications were made over the years, the most successful being that of Frederic Hewitt, one of the leaders of the London anaesthetic scene from the 1890s, who ingeniously enlarged the bellows tube so the narrower exit tube could travel inside it.

John Mann Crombie of the Cancer Hospital was a great advocate of chloroform. In 1873 he published a booklet recommending an inhaler of his own devising, for the self-administration of chloroform for pain or insomnia. The apparatus consisted of a face-piece connected by a tube to a bottle which was part-filled with chloroform. The patient squeezed a rubber bulb, which delivered the chloroform-laden air, and as drowsiness took over, so the pressure on the bulb relaxed. 'The inhalation of chloroform . . . is a most agreeable not to say delightful experience',[40] enthused Dr Crombie, who, one suspects, must have tested the apparatus extensively. 'As the administration proceeds there follow other feelings of a powerfully agreeable character . . . the respiratory sensations are extremely pleasurable.'[41]

The apparatus was not approved of by the profession, since it offered the public 'further opportunities for the abuse of anodynes.'[42] Crombie's penchant for self-medication was to be his downfall. In 1883, in considerable pain following an operation on an arm injury, he dosed himself from a bottle of morphine intended for injection, and died. He was thirty-nine.[43]

Scottish surgeons were unimpressed by the statistics. In 1876, G.H.B. MacLeod of the Western Infirmary, Glasgow, gave a lecture in which he reported that no surgical deaths had ever occurred either there or in the Royal Infirmary. 'True,' he added, 'four deaths have occurred from chloroform during that time in the latter institution, but they all took place when it was administered for comparatively trivial things in the ward.'[44] This mortality he dismissed as 'hardly worthy of computation'.[45]

Unable to disprove that ether was safer, he calmly waved the fact aside. 'This position might be, I think, strongly controverted if time allowed, but let it at present pass.'[46] This kind of teaching turned out doctors who believed that as long as a few simple rules were followed, the administration of chloroform was safe, and so few efforts were devoted to making it safer.

In England and on the continent, however, the belief that chloroform deaths arose from its action on the heart led to research to discover the mechanism by which this happened. Thomas (later Sir Thomas) Lauder Brunton, whose work on the effects of drugs upon the heart led to the use of amyl nitrate in the treatment of angina, was giving a great deal of thought to chloroform in 1875. He knew that stimulation of the vagus nerve slowed the action of the heart and theorised that low doses of chloroform irritated this nerve but abolished the reflex that countered it, whereas larger doses abolished both reactions. This work was to place him in a position of some eminence, and when, fourteen years later, his profession urgently needed an authority on the action of chloroform on the heart, Brunton was the man selected.

On the continent there were new developments in pre-medication. In the period between 1875 and 1880 important work was being carried out on the effects of giving atropine, a heart stimulant, before surgery under chloroform, but it took time for this to be accepted. In the UK there was considerable suspicion about combining powerful narcotic agents. English surgeons who were worried about the dangers of chloroform were more likely to turn to ether and nitrous oxide than give chloroform in conjunction with something else. In Scotland, of course, chloroform was safe and needed no pre-medication.

In 1880 the Glasgow committee, as it came to be known, finally published the results of its experiments, concluding that chloroform 'had a most disastrous action on the heart as well as upon the respiratory centre'.[47]

Ether was found superior to chloroform in every respect save one – it was slower. Following extensive trials of other anaesthetics the committee finally recommended 'ethidine dichloride', difficult to identify, but probably another highly dangerous solvent. The report had very little effect. Doctors who preferred ether because of its safety were undeterred by the extra few minutes required to apply it. Those who preferred chloroform continued to believe in it, and stated that the matter of its safety was still *sub judice*.

On the continent, chloroform continued its popularity, influenced by the work of Paul Bert, professor of physiology at the Sorbonne. In the early 1880s, he carried out a series of experiments with anaesthetics in which he established that the lethal dose was exactly double the anaesthetic dose. The interval between the two he called the '*zone maniable*'.[48] Measured in grams per 100 litres of air, the margin of safety for ether was 40 grams, but for chloroform only 12. Bert believed he was demonstrating a wholly new principle, which would make chloroform anaesthesia entirely safe. British journals pointed out that he was effectively travelling the same ground explored by Snow and Clover, with whose work he was unfamiliar,[49] but his work did have the effect of stimulating interest in the study of chloroform, and confidence that it could be made safe.

THE DANGER IN PURITY

From time to time it was suggested that the real reason behind chloroform deaths was impure chloroform, but the mechanism by which apparently 100 per cent pure chloroform would, after a time, develop impurities was obstinately obscure. Progress was hindered by the fact that there was not always complete communication between the surgeons, who insisted on absolute purity, the manufacturers, who wanted to preserve the product, and the chemists, who were trying to reconcile the previous two requirements.

There were numerous theories as to why chloroform decomposed, most of which blamed faults in the manufacturing process, which left chemical residues in the product. As late as 1871 an article in the *Pharmaceutical Journal* roundly ridiculed a German chemist who had observed that chloroform with added alcohol did not decompose. 'It would perhaps have been wiser if he had prided himself on the purity of his product instead of boasting of selling an adulterated article.'[50]

Alcohol had in fact been known to be a preservative of chloroform since as early as 1863, when it was used by David Rennie Brown of Macfarlan Smith,[51] but in the eagerness for a pure product it took many years for this to be appreciated. In 1881 a French chemist, Yvon, devised a test for purity so stringent that only the most freshly prepared chloroform could hope to pass it. A Dr Henry Brown complained[52] that this was pushing matters too far, as he had heard that alcohol was a preservative, and far less harmful than the products of decomposition. He later received a letter from Duncan and Flockhart, which confirmed what the manufacturers had known for years – that pure chloroform simply doesn't keep. 'The medical profession should not be dictated to by a French chemist who if he does not know, should have known that all acknowledged makers of chloroform be they French, German, American or English, add absolute alcohol to pure chloroform, so as to make it permanent',[53] said Brown, with some irritation.

The other matter, which had long been speculated upon was the nature of the decomposition products, which had been known to cause severe respiratory distress in both patients and medical staff. Hydrochloric acid had been identified early on, but by 1882 it was finally established that the action of light and air on chloroform also produced phosgene, which was later to earn notoriety as a poison gas in the First World War.[54]

THE 1880s

Joseph Clover's health had been steadily and inevitably declining. By 1882 he was too ill to work, and awaited the end with quiet resignation, slipping away in September aged fifty-seven. His death left the London anaesthesia scene bereft of a much needed guiding hand, and the next few years were a wilderness of confusion and conflict. By this time, the 'ether frenzy' was over. Deaths had occurred both under ether and nitrous oxide, and there was a renewal of interest in chloroform.

In the same year Joseph Lister experienced a chloroform death which must have been highly embarrassing.[55] He was then professor of surgery at King's College London and a healthy 27-year-old gentleman, terrified of chloroform, and presumably inspired by Lister's reputation for safety, made the trip from Manchester for the express purpose of having him perform an operation to open an abscess. Chloroform was applied, and the patient suddenly suffered what Lister described as 'an epilepiform fit' and died before the operation could commence. The death certificate, which gave the primary cause as the abscess and only secondarily the effects of chloroform, was taken to the district registrar, who declined to register and communicated with the coroner. The body was whisked away to Manchester for inquest. Lister was later obliged to admit that chloroform was the cause of death but insisted that it would have been just as likely to happen under any other anaesthetic. Lister's papers actually contain several accounts of deaths or near-deaths from chloroform, but he always attributed them to another cause, such as shock or heart disease. The death of the Manchester gentleman was the first in which his judgement had been questioned.

It may have been no coincidence that soon after this experience Lister modified his methods, adopting a similar procedure to the open-drop method advocated by Simpson some twenty years previously.

As the decade wore on, and deaths continued, debate hardened into immobility, the entrenched viewpoints of surgeons and anaesthetists preventing any progress on that front. Meanwhile, physiologists were making use of increasingly sophisticated devices for measuring functions such as heartbeat and respiration, and it seemed that the mystery of chloroform deaths would be solved not by observation of human patients, but laboratory experiments. Red herrings were to litter the path to certainty, and there were to be a number of disastrous wrong turnings before the answer was finally known.

ELEVEN

The Crime of Adelaide Bartlett

> Chloroform handed to her; chloroform in her possession; chloroform killing the man; the bottle of chloroform disappearing . . .
>
> *Mr Justice Wills, summing up*

In 1886 chloroform played a dominant role in a notorious murder trial, which both scandalised and titillated Victorian society.[1] An understanding of the unique properties of the fatal fluid were essential to the fate of the defendant, and can scarcely have been discussed publicly in such detail either before or since. In the dock was Adelaide Bartlett – young, attractive, mysterious; in the witness box, the Revd George Dyson, her admirer and dupe, an educated but callow and trusting Methodist minister; in the grave, Adelaide's husband, Edwin, a grocer whose most thrilling topic of conversation was the state of the provision trade. At the centre of it all, missing and never to be found, was a bottle of chloroform.

It is always a difficult task to disentangle the truth from rumour, error, speculation and downright lies, and never more so than here. Everything in Adelaide's history suggests that she was an accomplished liar, adept at manipulating others, especially men, to do her will, using every means at her disposal, from making herself into a wounded object of pity to shouting and stamping her foot.

Adelaide's mother was Clara Chamberlain, the daughter of a stock exchange clerk, who in 1853 married a Frenchman calling himself Adolphe de la Tremoille, and claiming to be the Comte de Thouars and son of the Duc de Thouars, also called Adolphe. This sounds very impressive, and presumably the Chamberlain family were impressed, but had they examined the family tree of the noble house of de la Tremoille they would have discovered that no one in that line bore the name of Adolphe. It seems very probable that Clara's husband was an impostor. In 1855 when Adelaide was born, her birth certificate reveals that the couple were living in rented accommodation in Orléans, where Adolphe was working as a teacher of mathematics.

One of the many myths surrounding Adelaide is that her wealthy father provided financial support, both for her early accommodation and her trial, but recently discovered evidence shows that by 1866 Adelaide was an orphan. In that year, Clara died of peritonitis in St Pancras Hospital on 14 November, aged just 33. The death certificate describes her as a widow. Adelaide and her younger sister, Clara, (called de Thouars in the 1871 census, and who was to die in January 1873), went to live with the family of Uncle William, her mother's brother, now something very substantial on the stock exchange.[2] This situation did not continue for long, and it seems that Adelaide created family tensions such that she was packed off to lodgings in Kingston upon Thames, where she took up residence with the family of Charles Bartlett. Another myth is that Adelaide's genteel accommodation was one of many properties owned by Charles. Yseult Bridges' classic work on this case[3] states that Charles was a well-to-do landlord, having married a widow of means, but official records not available when her book was written deny this. Charles Bartlett was a parcel carrier, who had married a draper's assistant, and their home was in a humble terraced house, in a district where the poorly paid inhabitants eked out their earnings by letting rooms.

Charles's brother Edwin was quite another matter, however. For one thing he was single, and the joint owner of a grocery business, which was clearly going places. He was an excellent catch. It was a short matter indeed for Adelaide to charm him, hinting that she had the expectation of a dowry from her wealthy uncle. There were only two obstacles to their marriage. One of these was Edwin's father, Edwin senior, a 57-year-old journeyman carpenter who did not welcome the match; but Edwin, at thirty, was his own man and would not let that stand in his way. The other problem was more difficult. Edwin and his partner, a Mr Baxter, had agreed to spend the first few years working hard to build up their trade, and this included a compact not to marry and set up households of their own, which would be a drain on finances. Edwin was currently living above one of the shops. Although only nineteen, Adelaide was able to manipulate things so that she got what she wanted. The wedding took place in April 1875, but she was sent to complete her schooling until such time as she and Edwin could set up home together, which was two years later. It seems that the promised dowry either never materialised or, if it did, was nothing like the amount Edwin had been led to expect.[4]

Living above the grocery store could hardly have been exciting, and in 1878 there was turmoil as Edwin senior accused Adelaide of an intrigue with Edwin's younger brother Frederick. Adelaide was said to have run away with Frederick, while her side of the story was that she had gone to stay with an aunt, wounded by her father-in-law's insulting accusations. Edwin's solution was to try and smooth over events and restore the even tenor of family life, and he persuaded his father to sign a document admitting that his accusations were false. The old man signed, grudgingly, but always maintained afterwards that he had only done so to keep the peace. Frederick had already dealt with the matter to his own satisfaction by running away to America.

In view of the shocking statements later made by Adelaide, it should be said at this point that there was never, in the early history of the Bartlett household, any suggestion that the marital relations of the couple were anything other than normal. It was unusual that having been married since 1875 Adelaide did not become pregnant until 1881, but it is possible that the marriage may not have been consummated until they cohabited, and we know from a witness at the trial that they used condoms. Edwin was a shrewd and ambitious man of business, and would have realised that the key to prosperity lay not only in hard work and sound knowledge of his trade, but in limiting the size of his family. The child was stillborn, and in the remaining four years of the Bartlett marriage, there were no further pregnancies.

In 1884 the couple were finally able to leave their accommodation over the shop, and found a delightful cottage in the village of Merton Abbey, where the nearby railway station would take Edwin to his work each morning. Adelaide seemed to have few interests, apart from reading and embroidery, and spent time helping the daily maid with a little light housework, and looking after the kennel of St Bernard dogs which were Edwin's only hobby. There were few visitors, the only recorded ones being George and Alice Mathews, friends from London, and Annie Walker, the midwife who had befriended Adelaide while staying to care for her after the birth of her child.

If Adelaide was discontented, there were no outward signs, and if she was bored, there was no alternative to stimulate her. Edwin worked long hours at the shop, and at home seemed contented enough as long as he had a good dinner, but he was adept at papering over cracks. From comments he made later it seems that Adelaide was not happy, and the sexual side of the marriage had deteriorated. Part of this may have been due to the state of Edwin's teeth. Some years previously he had had most of his teeth sawn off at gum level so a false set could be fitted, but this had irritated his mouth so much he had given up not only the false teeth but his toothbrush. What remained were spongy gums and rotting stumps surrounded by masses of decaying food. His only relief was rubbing the gums with chlorodyne.

It was a situation that only required a catalyst to set off a fatal train of events, and in 1884 it arrived in the unlikely form of George Dyson, the 26-year-old probationer Methodist minister who had recently taken charge of the tiny chapel at Merton. George was by Bartlett standards very well educated, and was currently completing an external degree course at Trinity College, Dublin. His aim in life was to be useful and entertaining, and in an age where conversation was a valued art, he made a great effort to be an amusing and interesting companion, able to talk on a wide variety of subjects. One of the many things he introduced into discussion was the fashionable interest in hypnotism. It was not a subject Edwin had any particular interest in, but Adelaide clearly recalled the conversation and later put it to good use.

George's pastoral visits lit up the dull Bartlett household and he soon became a frequent visitor. Although Adelaide later claimed it was Edwin's wish that she should be educated, it may well have been she who suggested that the young minister should give her lessons in subjects such as history, Latin and Greek. George saw her at home and sometimes at his lodgings and they often took lunch together, or went for walks. It was not long before George was thoroughly smitten by the lovely Adelaide. For his part, Edwin, trusting the man of the cloth, was delighted to find that his wife was a much better and happier woman since the minister entered their lives. It was about this time that Adelaide began to urge Edwin to change his will. Made before the Married Women's Property Act, which gave married women greater control over their property, it left everything to Adelaide on condition she did not remarry. This, as Adelaide told Annie Walker in front of Edwin, was unfair.

The summer of 1885 was idyllic, but it could not last forever, and George was offered a better post at a chapel in Putney, to commence at the start of September. By now he had become an essential in their lives. The house in Merton was given up, and the Bartletts moved to an apartment on the first floor of a house in Claverton Street, Pimlico, near Victoria station, which was convenient both for Edwin's work and George's visits. There was another change in the household arrangements – for the first time in the marriage the Bartletts occupied separate beds.

By this time, George was a greatly troubled young man, for his adoration of Adelaide was occupying his thoughts so much that it was distracting him from his work. She was not only a married woman, but also the wife of a close friend for whom he had the highest regard. George, who was a decent man, decided to do the decent thing. That September he had been astonished when Edwin informed him that he had made a new will and had named him as an executor. Embarrassed, George confessed his admiration for Adelaide and the fact that he had been thinking of not seeing the couple so frequently. To his amazement Edwin seemed untroubled by this, and expressed his confidence in and regard for the young minister, urging him to continue the friendship that had been so beneficial to Adelaide. Still, George was concerned, and it is probable that Edwin discussed the matter with Adelaide, for at George's very first visit to the Pimlico apartments she told him a manifestly untrue story which was to put their relationship on a completely different footing.

Edwin, she said, was suffering from a serious internal disease, and probably had no more than a year to live. When George asked if Edwin had seen a doctor Adelaide said that she had consulted a Dr Nichols on his behalf, who had both diagnosed and treated the patient without even having seen him. Dr Nichols was no figment of the imagination, but the American author of a book on healthy living, which, dealing as it did with the morality of relationships, birth control (for which it advised abstinence) and natural childbirth, was not something the average householder would have left lying around.[5] Adelaide, who took an interest in medical subjects, had a copy of the book, and had even lent it to Mr Mathews, who later became very embarrassed by the subject and asserted that he had handed it back unread. Adelaide had never met Dr Nichols, but in 1881 she had written to his wife for advice and it was through her that the nurse had been sent to attend Adelaide for the birth of her child. The Nicholses did not believe in using pain-killers for childbirth, assuring expectant mothers that if they lived healthily, they would not require to be made 'dead drunk' on chloroform and the like. Mary Gove Nichols was also a writer on health matters, and was convinced that she had the ability to heal by touch.[6] Having experienced an unhappy first marriage, Mary avowed that a union without love was tantamount to prostitution, while a loving relationship, even without legal sanction, was a true marriage, a concept Adelaide had no difficulty in taking on board.

Adelaide's obvious knowledge of the Nicholses' work was enough to convince George that she had indeed consulted a doctor. She implored him, however, not to discuss Edwin's illness with him as it was a matter about which he was very sensitive. George agreed. She assured him that she knew a great deal about medicines, and owned a medicine chest, so was capable of dealing with the symptoms of Edwin's illness when they arose.

There was no more talk of George breaking off the relationship with the Bartletts. Apart from the desire to be useful to them, and be there when they needed him most, the thought was forming at the back of his mind that after Edwin's death, when a decent interval had passed, he could eventually marry the lovely widow. The frequency of his visits increased, and there was one occasion when Alice Fulcher, the maid, entered the drawing room to find George sitting on the floor at Adelaide's feet, his head in her lap.

Edwin was actually in good health, and had suffered very few illnesses requiring medical attention. George could see no obvious signs of fatal disease, only that Edwin was tired after a long day at work, and sometimes had indigestion, which was not surprising in a man who spent his day tasting cheese and butter, and was unable to chew his food.

In November 1885 Edwin suddenly became very ill, with violent vomiting and diarrhoea and stomach pain. In a state of collapse, he took to his bed, where he was a very depressed patient, and Adelaide went to fetch the local doctor. Dr Alfred Leach, whose surgery was just a few minutes walk away, could not have been better chosen. Twenty-nine years of age, confident and arrogant, with an enormous sense of his own professional status, he was also naturally inclined to accept on trust everything that Adelaide told him. He was a man who loved to form a theory, but having done so, could not be shaken from it.

On examining Edwin he noticed an unusual symptom, a blue line around the margin of his gums. With suspicion growing in his mind he hurried back to consult his textbooks and confirmed that this was a sign of poisoning with some heavy metallic element such as mercury or lead. Mercury compounds were a common treatment for venereal disease, and Leach formed the theory that Edwin had been taking it for this reason, omitting to tell his trusting wife. Returning to Edwin, he took the attitude that he at least wasn't going to be fooled, but to his surprise Edwin denied that he had ever had such a disease, much less taken mercury for it. An examination revealed no sign of any problems in that area. There was then some discussion of Edwin's sex life, which Leach later skated around with irritating delicacy when he wrote about the case,[7] but the general tenor of the conversation suggested that there was not a great deal of sexual activity in the Bartlett household, that Edwin had normal appetites and satisfied them without either being unfaithful or indulging in solitary vices – how was not indicated. Leach's next theory was that Edwin had a peculiar idiosyncrasy for mercury, having taken a small amount in a single pill he admitted swallowing, and this had reacted with the salts in his rotted teeth to cause the blue line.

Edwin's father was most anxious about his son's illness, which he became aware of when visiting the grocery shop. Adelaide, who did not want the old man interfering or calling in another doctor, denied him entry to the house as often as she could, just sending him the occasional curt note with a progress report. One longer missive showed that his accusations of 1878 still rankled:

Sunday night

Dear Mr Bartlett
I hear that you are a little disturbed because Edwin has been too ill to see you. I wish, if possible to be friends with you, but you must place yourself on the same footing as other persons – that is to say, you are welcome here when I invite you, and at no other time. You seem to forget that I have not been in bed for thirteen days, and consequently am too tired to speak to visitors. I am sorry to speak so plainly, but I wish you to understand that I have neither forgotten nor forgiven the past. Edwin will be pleased to see you on Monday evening any time after six.

Eventually, Edwin was on the mend, which Dr Leach attributed to his treatment, but which may very well have been due to the fact that Adelaide was no longer poisoning him. Only then was Edwin senior permitted to visit, and a second doctor was called, who formed the opinion that Edwin was a hypochondriac, declared him to be a well man and said he should get up and go out.

Edwin, however, was curiously disinclined to go out, and was most resistant to Leach's suggestion that he no longer needed a doctor. Just as it seemed that he was yielding to Leach's persuasion to take a trip to the seaside, Edwin had a terrible shock – a worm was found in his faeces. This created a nervous relapse. Leach spent a day going back and forth between his surgery and the Bartlett home, supplying medication. There was a worm powder called santonin, which after taking had to be cleared from the system with laxatives. Not only did the laxatives seem to have no effect at all, but Edwin exhibited none of the unpleasant symptoms of having santonin remaining in his system. Leach went home, shaking his head at this unusual patient, but the most likely explanation is that Adelaide, who had control over the medication taken by her husband, gave him something other than santonin and laxatives. If, as one might speculate, the worm was not passed by Edwin, but procured by Adelaide from the kennels and planted, then she would have been concerned that laxatives would reveal there to have been no worm infestation at all. (No sign of worms was found at Edwin's post-mortem.)

Towards the end of December Edwin made a startling statement to Leach, in which he said he thought he had been hypnotised by a good friend, and he and his wife had been doing things beyond all reason. What these things were he did not say, but in a later conversation he admitted standing over the sleeping form of his wife holding his hands over her to try and draw the energy from her body. It seems as if Adelaide and Edwin had been carrying out experiments in animal magnetism, and Edwin, convinced that he was able to draw strength from Adelaide, and also possibly from Leach, was in a highly nervous state and felt dependent on them both.

There is no proof, of course, that Adelaide was poisoning Edwin, but she had exhibited some of the classic behaviour of the poisoner. She had primed George by announcing that Edwin would die, even before he was ill, invented a mysterious internal complaint, taken charge of all the sick-room arrangements, and tended him constantly to the point of sleeping in a chair beside his bed. She had restricted access from his father and obstructed attempts to call in a second doctor until the symptoms abated. A situation had also been created where Edwin was effectively under her control, afraid to leave the house, with a strong sense of dependence on her presence.

As the year drew to a close, Edwin was feeling much improved, and while he still implored Leach to visit he was looking forward to getting back to his business. Leach had even persuaded him to go on a short drive and had also arranged for Edwin to visit the local dentist and have his remaining bad teeth and the rotting stumps removed, the gums being painted with a solution of cocaine. His only remaining health problem was persistent insomnia. On 31 December, Edwin, relaxing after his most recent visit to the dentist, was enjoying a brief visit from his landlady Mrs Doggett, when Adelaide suddenly asked her if she had ever taken chloroform, and if so, was it a nice or pleasant feeling? Startled, Mrs Doggett said she had, but couldn't remember anything about it.

There was already a bottle of chloroform in the house. On 28 December, Adelaide and George had gone out for a stroll on the Embankment, and she had asked him if he would buy a bottle of chloroform for her. She explained that she needed it for Edwin, but did not think the chemist would sell it to her. Edwin, she said, had terrible paroxysms, which were a symptom of his fatal disease, and the only thing that soothed him was chloroform. She was skilled in using it and had employed it many times before for that purpose. It had previously been obtained for her by Annie Walker the nurse, but Annie was now in America. This entire story, as Adelaide later admitted, was a pack of lies, but George swallowed it.

Adelaide had asked for a medicine bottle full of chloroform, but when George tried to buy chloroform he discovered that only very tiny bottles were available, and he purchased three, all from shops where he was known by sight. When buying the chloroform he told the chemists he required it for cleaning clothes, for having believed the story Adelaide had told him he must have seen that without the lady's lovely presence it sounded unconvincing. He later borrowed a medicine bottle from his landlady and poured the contents of the three small bottles into it. This he gave to Adelaide.

On 31 December 1885, Edwin and Adelaide retired for the night, Edwin in the little bed he had occupied in the front parlour since his illness, Adelaide in the chair beside him. What happened in the next few hours are the very heart of the mystery.

At 4 a.m. on 1 January 1886 Adelaide went upstairs to knock on the door of Alice Fulcher the maidservant. Rousing her from her bed she told her that Edwin was dead and she must go and fetch Dr Leach at once. Leaving Alice hurriedly dressing, Adelaide then knocked on the door of the Doggetts' bedroom with the same story. Mr Frederick Doggett was a registrar of births, marriages and deaths. It was his critical eye that was therefore the first that was passed over the Bartlett apartments after Edwin's death. As soon as he entered the room Doggett noticed something very unusual, a sweetish smell that seemed to be very reminiscent of chloric ether – the solution of chloroform in alcohol. There was a scent of it coming from a partly full brandy glass on the mantelpiece and also from the fluid sprinkled on the chest of the corpse. Edwin was dead – there was no doubt about that – and the temperature of the body suggested he had been dead for some hours.

When Leach arrived, he and Doggett examined the contents of the room, but nothing was found which could have contributed to death – certainly there was no bottle of chloroform. Adelaide could only say that she had been asleep by Edwin's side, holding his foot, and all had seemed well. She had awoken with a cramp in her arm, and found the body face down. She had turned him over, sprinkled brandy on his chest, and poured a considerable amount down his throat, but to no avail, whereupon she had immediately gone for help. There were several things wrong with this account. The difference in temperature between the upper and lower surfaces of the body showed that it had never been on its front. It was impossible to pour substantial amounts of brandy down the throat of a corpse, and if Adelaide had at once run for help, why was it that the parlour fire looked as though it had been recently tended?

Edwin senior, called to see the body, at once expressed his suspicions, demanded a post-mortem and engaged his own medical specialist. The body was moved into the back bedroom, and in the subsequent clearing-up the half-full brandy glass, probably the most important clue in the case, was taken downstairs and washed.

When the examination was carried out on 2 January, five doctors, including Leach, attended. Downstairs in the smoking-room, George, Adelaide and the Bartlett solicitor Mr Wood waited for the result, with Edwin senior pacing up and down on the pavement outside. As soon as the eminent Dr Green had dashed away in his carriage, Edwin senior went in, and after a while Dr Leach came downstairs and summoned everyone upstairs. As they stood at the foot of the stairs, Adelaide turned to her loathed father-in-law and assured him comfortingly that she would look after him exactly as if Edwin was alive. As they walked up, Dr Leach was unable to resist making his contribution. They had, he told George, noticed the smell of chloroform in the stomach contents but he believed Dr Green was mistaken and it was only due to the chlorodyne that Edwin used on his gums. George must have been thunderstruck.

In the drawing room, it was announced that the contents of the stomach were suspicious and had been preserved for further examination. It was necessary for Adelaide to leave the house at once, and the rooms would have to be sealed until the coroner had finished with them, Dr Leach having charge of the keys. Adelaide asked to be allowed to take her hat, which was in the back bedroom, but she was not permitted to go in; instead, Dr Leach brought the drawer which contained her hat and she removed it. George accompanied her to the home of the Mathews, and on the way asked her what had become of the bottle of chloroform he had bought for her. To his surprise she snapped at him that he was not to trouble her at this critical time.

Back home, poor George had a sleepless night. The fate of the bottle of chloroform haunted him. If it should be shown that it had been responsible for Edwin's death, then he knew that his career was in ruins. The following day was a Sunday, and George Dyson was due to preach at the local chapel. His journey there included a walk across Tooting Bec common, and on the way he threw away the three small bottles that had contained the chloroform.

On the Monday he went to see Adelaide and this time challenged her outright about the fate of the bottle of chloroform. A fine row ensued, in which she stamped up and down the room, and demanded to know if he suspected her of murder.

'You did tell me that Edwin was going to die soon!' exclaimed George, just as Alice Mathews entered the room.

'No I did not!' Adelaide replied.

In that terrible thunderclap of a moment, George Dyson knew that he had been duped, and realised that all the stories Adelaide had told him had been false. He bent his head on the piano and said, 'Oh my God!'

After a few moments of silence, Alice said quietly, 'Don't you think you had better go?'

He went, but his parting words were, 'I am a ruined man!'

When Alice asked for an explanation of the scene Adelaide could only say lamely that George had been asking for the return of a poem he had given her.

George was still determined to carry out his duties as an executor, although he returned to Adelaide Edwin's gold watch she had given him on 2 January and repaid some money he owed. On 6 January, Adelaide and Alice set out in freezing conditions for Claverton Street, as Adelaide had heard from the solicitor that it was now possible to recover her possessions. George arrived to deliver some letters and they set out together. On the way their train passed by Peckham Rye pond, which was frozen over. At Victoria station Adelaide sent George to buy some cord to tie up her boxes and the two ladies went to Dr Leach's house to collect the keys. Leach was out, but the ladies declined to wait and went on to Claverton Street. Despite the fact that the rooms were supposed to have been sealed, they were admitted, probably by Alice Fulcher, and set about packing up Adelaide's possessions. When George had finished buying the cord he arrived at Dr Leach's, was given the keys and proceeded to Claverton Street, where Mr Doggett's father let him in and made him wait in the hall.

When the ladies emerged, George handed Adelaide the keys and they returned to Dr Leach's, as that gentleman had wished to talk to Adelaide. In the waiting room, over tea, George asked Alice about Edwin's health, and discovered what he had by then suspected, that his dead friend had never had a serious illness. Following her conversation with Dr Leach, Adelaide returned alone to Claverton Street, the key to the back bedroom drawer now safely in her possession.

On the following day the inquest opened and was adjourned. George and Adelaide had a meeting in a tea-house afterwards, and he again broached the subject of the chloroform bottle. He said he was prepared to tell the truth, but Adelaide had a simpler solution – if he did not incriminate her, then she would not incriminate him. He was unable to countenance this request, and they parted coldly. By now, George had confessed all to both Alice and George Mathews, and on 9 January in a meeting at their house he challenged Adelaide to tell him what had happened to the chloroform bottle. Insisting that she had never opened or used it, she told him that she had collected it from Claverton Street on 6 January, and on the way home had poured the contents out of the train window and thrown the bottle into Peckham Rye pond. George's only hope of salvation, a sealed bottle containing the full amount of chloroform he had purchased, proving that it could not have been the cause of Edwin's death, was lost forever. He left the house shortly afterwards, and never spoke to Adelaide again.

Alice Mathews was now well aware that Adelaide had been telling lies both to her and George, and forced her to admit it. It can be no coincidence that two days later Adelaide moved to lodgings. Over the next few days, careful analysis of Edwin's stomach contents confirmed that he had died from drinking liquid chloroform, the estimate being that he had consumed about an ounce. Apart from the chloroform, his stomach contained only the remains of his last meal. Of alcohol there was only the merest trace. When Edwin had taken his dose of chloroform, he had swallowed it neat.

On 18 January George decided finally to tell the whole story to a fellow minister and on his advice consulted a solicitor. Things were now looking serious for Adelaide, and she was well aware that she would soon have some explaining to do. Dr Leach had made an appointment to see her on 26 January to discuss the results of the analysis, and when she arrived it was with a carefully crafted story. The tale she told was so extraordinary and in parts so ridiculous that Leach, excited at being given this vital information, swelled with importance and believed it all. In time, the public believed it too. According to Adelaide she had been married at sixteen (she had been nineteen) and because of Edwin's 'strange ideas' it was agreed that it would be a marriage of companionship only. There had only ever been one act of intercourse, that which resulted in the pregnancy. Edwin, she said, had surrounded her with male admirers and enjoyed their appreciation of her, but she had found this a sore trial. When they met George Dyson, Edwin had thrown them together, instructed her to kiss him, and eventually given her to the young minister as his affianced wife. Then came the twist in the tale – after years of neglect, after giving her to another man, and, moreover, while lying on a bed of sickness, Edwin had suddenly decided to claim his marital rights. In a stupendous piece of double-think, Adelaide explained that she could not agree to this as she had been given to Mr Dyson and could not be unfaithful to him. In an era when the faithless wife was beyond the pale, she had cleverly converted her intrigue with George into the real marriage to which she had to remain true.

In order to prevent Edwin's unwanted attentions, Adelaide said she had obtained the chloroform with the idea of sprinkling it on a handkerchief and waving it in his face whenever occasion demanded. She had later regretted this and one night had placed the bottle into Edwin's hands and told him why she had bought it. As to the fate of the bottle, she insisted that when Leach and Doggett searched the room it was there on the mantelpiece. It was the one point in her story which Leach was never able to resolve to his satisfaction.

Inevitably, Adelaide was arrested and charged with the murder of her husband, and, to his distress, George Dyson was also charged, though on the first day of the trial he was released, no case being made against him. His appearance in the witness box, giving evidence against the woman he had once loved, evoked a great deal of sympathy for her.

Adelaide was extraordinarily fortunate in her choice of defence counsel. Sir Edward Clarke, master of the moving speech, already had a reputation for winning difficult cases. Following the death of his first wife from tuberculosis, a pale, fragile-looking woman in need of his help was sure to win his sympathy. He saw at once that the trial promised to be one of the great cases of the decade, and that chloroform and its properties was crucial to the outcome. He at once dropped all his other work, and devoted his efforts to this one case, spending a great deal of time studying medical books. Sir Charles Russell, the Attorney General, a no less able man, who undertook the prosecution, was by contrast heavily involved in parliamentary matters, and was not able to devote so much time to the case. While Clarke took pains to be always present in court, Russell was absent much of the time, leaving a great deal of the questioning to his juniors.

There were only three possible ways Edwin could have died – accidental overdose, suicide or murder. From the outset the prosecution theory, that Adelaide had first rendered Edwin unconscious with inhaled chloroform as he slept then poured the liquid down his throat, was fraught with problems. Clarke was easily able to produce a great deal of medical evidence to show that chloroforming someone in their sleep had only ever been consistently successful with children. Even if Adelaide, with no experience of the matter, had been able to chloroform Edwin, she would have had to be able to judge the exact stage of narcosis when analgesia prevented the pain attendant on swallowing the liquid, while at the same time the swallowing reflex was still present. Clarke successfully represented to the jury that an operation of this delicacy was impossible for the lay person to achieve. He was probably correct. In any case, the whole prosecution story was destroyed by questions placed not by either counsel but by the foreman of the jury to Dr Thomas Stevenson, the medical expert who had analysed the remains.

These questions elicited the opinion that if chloroform was administered to a sleeping person, some of it might stay in the mouth, or remain at the upper part of the windpipe, creating irritation of the membranes. If a person in a seated position had drunk it down quickly, however, it would pass rapidly over the inner surfaces of the throat, and there would be no irritation at all. Since the post-mortem had not found any such irritation, the conclusion was obvious. When Edwin had drunk the chloroform he had been sitting up.

Not that the trial went entirely Adelaide's way. Condoms had been found in Edwin's trouser pockets, and Annie Walker testified that both Adelaide and Edwin had told her the pregnancy was the result not of their only act of intercourse but their only unprotected act. This effectively demolished the fable of the celibate marriage. By this time, however, the trial was won. Adelaide, as described in virtually every newspaper report of the trial, had spent the entire time sitting motionless in the dock, her body drooping in a pose that suggested abject abandonment. The hearts of the solid gentlemen of the jury were moved. Clarke called no witnesses for the defence, thus denying Russell the chance to use his greatest skill, cross-examination, while the eloquent closing speech for the defence brought tears to the eyes. Adelaide was acquitted to a great uproar of applause.

This leaves the all-important question – how did she do it?

Nothing in Edwin's demeanour suggests for a moment that he would have committed suicide. He had been a miserable patient, but he was on the mend and looking forward to getting back to work. The only other possibility was that he had swallowed the chloroform as a sleeping draught and simply overestimated the amount. But Adelaide cannot have been more than a few yards away from him when this happened, even if she had gone into the back bedroom to wash at the hand basin. If Edwin had swallowed an overdose by accident he would have appreciated his terrible error almost immediately, and there would have been several minutes when he was able to call out for assistance before he became unconscious. Given Adelaide's highly suspicious behaviour, the equation can only add up to murder.

The prosecution failed to prove murder mainly because it pinned its hopes on a theory that was ultimately too complex. In the Bartlett household there was a medical book which was produced in evidence at the trial – *Squire's Companion to the British Pharmacopoeia*. This lists a number of medicines alphabetically, and whatever knowledge of chloroform Adelaide had probably came almost entirely from the pages of this book. Here Adelaide would have learned that chloroform 'evaporates speedily, and leaves no residue and no unpleasant odour',[8] and that 'mixed with strong spirits, camphor liniment, soap liniment, olive oil, oil of turpentine, it dissolves perfectly'.[9] Medicinally it could be given internally as 'a sedative narcotic and anti-spasmodic',[10] the dose being 'one to five minims, with yolk of egg and mucilage, in syrup or in a teaspoonful of brandy',[11] while 10–20 minims of chloric ether are 'frequently prescribed to give a sweetness to draughts and to cover nauseous flavours'.[12]

In other words, it was a sweet-tasting narcotic, which dissolved in alcohol and would evaporate without trace. There is no mention in the book of the fiery burning taste of pure liquid chloroform, no mention of the consequences of a large dose, of irritation to the stomach, pain and vomiting. Nowhere did the book give an indication of what the fatal dose might be. When Adelaide gave Edwin the chloroform she did not know what the fatal dose was, but given the amount of the therapeutic dose she must have realised that an ounce was not exactly going to do him good.

We cannot doubt that Adelaide read the book: at the inquest[13] it was brought into court, where the coroner observed not only that it fell open at the page for chloroform but there was a note on the page – what sort he did not reveal. Her reasons for choosing chloroform as a means of murder are clear enough in the light of Edwin's earlier poisoning which had left the telltale blue line around the gums. Here, it must have seemed, was something that would evaporate leaving no trace of its action. It did not occur to her that it would remain in liquid form in the stomach.

Adelaide's original plan may well have been to administer the chloroform mixed with brandy, persuading Edwin that it was a sleeping draught. There was no brandy in the house, as Edwin was not a great drinker of spirits, but on 30 December Adelaide wrote to Mr Baxter asking him to bring round a bottle from the shop. If she had tried the experiment of mixing chloroform and brandy she would have been surprised to find that instead of the two liquids combining, they quickly separate into two quite distinct layers. Another plan was required, and here Adelaide fell back on her old techniques of persuasion. She began by mentioning chloroform to Mrs Doggett in front of Edwin, representing that it was a pleasant item to take, in much the same way as she had aired her dissatisfaction about the will in front of Annie Walker. Once Edwin had agreed to take the chloroform it was just a matter of pouring the dose into the brandy glass and handing it to him with the suggestion that he knock it back quickly. It was as simple as that. Of course, he would have choked at once, and maybe this was the moment when the brandy was splashed into the glass and handed to him, but he probably wanted a drink of water instead. The glass, mainly brandy with a little chloroform below it, was placed on the mantelpiece and forgotten. Gradually, Edwin became unconscious, and began to snore.

Perhaps Adelaide had not intended him to die that night. She had needed to do something for he had been talking of making a regular allowance to her father-in-law in the new year. Not realising that chloroform, unlike lead or mercury, is not a cumulative poison she may have envisaged a slow decline, with Edwin in a dreamy state most of the time. Adelaide had said that she slept between the hours of 12 and 4 a.m., and this seems very likely, as there is no evidence that she took so much as a nap on the following day. Awaking at four, she tended the fire and only then saw that Edwin was dead. She splashed him with a little brandy as evidence of her frantic efforts at revival and then hurried upstairs for the greatest performance of her life.

Chloroform left alone in a glass will evaporate very quickly. The combination of brandy and chloroform in a glass produces an interesting effect – protected by the floating layer of the much lighter brandy, the chloroform does not evaporate rapidly, but a combined vapour of chloroform and alcohol seeps into the air, and after about thirty minutes, someone entering the room is immediately aware of a sweetish smell.[14] The scent that Mr Doggett identified as chloric ether as he walked into the Bartletts' drawing room was probably the combination of chloroform and brandy, which had been permeating through the room for the last four hours, and to which Adelaide, who had been in the room, would have become desensitised. It cannot have been recent, for if she had, as she said, poured out the brandy immediately before summoning Mr Doggett, there would have been no time for the smell to fill the room.

One more question remains – what happened to the bottle of chloroform?

With hindsight, she should of course have disposed of it immediately, but she did not. If she had, as she thought, committed the perfect murder with an untraceable poison, there was no reason to throw it away; also there would have been quite a bit left in the bottle, just handy for her next victim, who would undoubtedly have been Edwin senior. When she was removed from the house on 2 January, she had no opportunity to retrieve the bottle. It had probably been put in the drawer in the back room, and she had tried to get there on the pretext of fetching her hat. Adelaide's agitated reactions to George's questioning up to 6 January show that that she was a very frightened woman. Was it conceivable that the bottle did remain there until 6 January? Dr Leach said that he had not searched the drawers in the back room, and when the coroner's officer was sent to get the specimens for analysis he too did not make a search but simply brought away the bottles and packages he had been asked to fetch. The official police search of the premises was not made until 11 January, after Adelaide's visit.

On 7 January Adelaide's talk with George after the inquest reveals her in a much more relaxed and confident mood. It is very probable therefore that she did indeed get the bottle on 6 January and, as she had described, empty the contents out of the train window, tossing the bottle out afterwards. Not into Peckham Rye pond, which was frozen over, but by then it would have been too dark to see where she was throwing it. The pond story was just a dramatic flourish.

There are two stories told of Adelaide's activities after the trial, and neither stands up to examination. Yseult Bridges, in the second edition of her book, tells of how Adelaide became involved in fund-raising during the First World War, and gives a very detailed and convincing story of a Madame Bartlett making speeches and taking supplies across the channel to hospitals in France. This story is quite true, and a Mme Bartlett did all of these things, but she was Caroline Gardner Bartlett, an American opera singer, not Adelaide.[15]

Kate Clarke[16] published a photograph of some American nurses aboard the hospital ship *Maine* in 1899, one of whom bears a strong resemblance to Adelaide. Clarke claims that this was indeed Adelaide, that she had changed her name to Barbara McBean, and was making trouble on board. An article[17] and photograph[18] in the *Nursing Record* identify this nurse as a Miss McVean, who qualified at Bellevue Hospital, New York, in 1898, and her first name, according to the hospital archives, was Sarah.[19] None of the American nurses were called Barbara, or indeed McBean, although Lady Randolph Churchill, who organised the venture, did write in an undated letter of a disruptive nurse called Barbara.[20] In her reminiscences, however, she mentions a contingent of nurses taken on at Cape Town who were badly behaved, so presumably Barbara was one of these.[21] Could Adelaide have been Sarah McVean? The archives of Bellevue Hospital show that Sarah McVean was born in New York in 1873, making her twenty-six years old in 1899. Adelaide would have been forty-four. In 1885, when Adelaide was in England, the Bellevue records show that Sarah was in America suffering from diphtheria. Adelaide was not Sarah McVean.

Adelaide disappears from history with Edwin's £4,000 in her pocket, her fate unknown. George Dyson's later history is also unknown, although he is reputed to have emigrated to Australia. He must have wanted to make absolutely sure he never bumped into Adelaide again.

TWELVE

THE SLEEP OF DEATH

> I got the towel and sponge, made the towel into a cone shape, and saturated the sponge with chloroform. I tried it on my own face and got a strong effect. Then I put it over Mr Rice's face and ran out. . . . In about half an hour, I went back . . .
>
> *Statement of Charles Jones, April 1901*[1]

In the summer of 1855, Brigadier General W.S. Harney, a veteran of the United States–Mexico war, marched west from Kansas with a force of 600 men. His object was to ensure the safety of settlers moving along the Oregon Trail to California by impressing the marauding Sioux with the power of the white man. Harney's massacre of a Sioux encampment in September was a devastating move, and when he called a council at Fort Pierre in March 1856 most of the headmen attended. In demonstrating his superiority he had more than just bullets in his arsenal – he called upon the potent magic of chloroform. Harney told the assembled chiefs that he could kill a man and then restore him to life. He then ordered a surgeon to demonstrate this miracle. Fortunately the subject was a dog. The surgeon duly applied chloroform, and the limp form of the animal was passed around the chiefs so they could confirm it had expired. They nodded and agreed that the dog was 'plenty dead'. Harney then ordered the surgeon to bring the dog back to life. The Sioux had been correct, however, for the dog had gone the way of Professor Brande's guinea-pig, and was indeed, to Harney's embarrassment and the chiefs' amusement, 'plenty dead'.[2]

Correspondence and visits exchanged between doctors in the UK and their transatlantic brethren, especially in Boston, led some British doctors to believe that chloroform was little used in the United States, but this was not the case. The qualities of chloroform that made it so useful on the battlefield were also a boon in the remoter regions of the American west. Boston remained the home of ether, and influenced the neighbouring cities of New York, Philadelphia and Baltimore. But chloroform was not unknown in the North-eastern states, and from time to time there were reports of fatal accidents there, either from chloroform or ether/chloroform mixtures, when a hapless dentist could only claim, without any fear of contradiction, that he had given it because the patient had insisted upon it. In other parts of the USA, chloroform and ether were both employed, while the Southern states followed the French model, and used chloroform almost exclusively.

American journalists liked a chloroform story as much as their European counterparts. One newspaper declared that two ladies had been found unconscious on the ground after being robbed of their jewellery while drugged by chloroform. Houses were frequently said to have been robbed after their inmates were rendered unconscious, and once it was claimed that the customers in a store had had their pockets picked after the air had been so impregnated with chloroform that they were unaware of what was happening.[3] A Dr Stephen Rogers of New York concluded, as Dr Snow had done, that given the length of time it took to produce insensibility, the resistance of the person being attacked with chloroform would add to rather than diminish the difficulties of the thief.[4]

DEAD DRUNK

One of the most prolific users of chloroform was Herman Webster Mudgett, who went under a number of names during his criminal career, the best-known being Henry Howard Holmes.[5] Born in 1860, Holmes had trained as a doctor, but he soon turned to a life of crime. In 1894 he succeeded in committing a murder by both inhalation and ingestion of chloroform, leaving no real clues as to how he had achieved it.

Holmes was a serial bigamist and fraudster, and an emotionless murderer of men, women and children. Manipulative, plausible, and resourceful, he had the ability to devise horrors that were the stuff of nightmares, and make them into solid fact. His unique achievement was to design and build a sprawling three-storey hotel in Chicago whose maze-like construction, multiple rooms, twisting corridors and secret passages were like something from the most lurid kind of Gothic novel. Since he hired and fired about 500 workmen during the two years it took to complete, the only person who knew all the secrets of the building's layout was himself. At street level, there was a row of shops, some run by Holmes, some leased. The two upper floors were mainly bedrooms. Many of the visitors spent their last nights there, killed by the gas that Holmes piped to their rooms. He was also said to be adept at using chloroform, though there is no actual evidence that he had invented a foolproof way of chloroforming sleeping adults. His main motives were profit, and the elimination of discarded mistresses. Disposal of the bodies was no problem, for the basement was supplied with vats of acid and quicklime, and dissecting tables.

One of the construction workers hired by Holmes stayed on long after the Castle, as it came to be known, was completed in 1890. He was Benjamin Freelon Pitezel, who had become a willing associate of Holmes in his crooked business deals. Tall and muscular, his once good looks had been eroded by alcoholism, and bar fights had left him with a broken nose and missing teeth. He was devoted to his wife Carrie and their five children.

Late in 1893, as his many creditors finally closed in, Holmes left Chicago, and he and Pitezel arrived in the South, where they began a number of fraudulent enterprises, moving from city to city to escape prosecution by their victims. It was in St Louis, in July 1894, that something happened which Holmes had never anticipated – he was arrested and jailed. It took ten days to effect a release on bail but in that time he managed to complete his plans for an insurance swindle he had been planning for some time.

Back in November of 1893 Holmes had arranged for a policy of $10,000 on the life on Benjamin Pitezel. The plan was, as he explained to his accomplice, that after a few months a disfigured corpse, which Holmes would procure, would be identified as Pitezel, he would collect the money and they would split it equally. Seeing a chance to establish financial security for his family, Pitezel agreed. The one thing lacking in the whole scheme was the services of a crooked lawyer. While in jail, Holmes got talking to an armed robber called Marion Hedgepeth, who was able to recommend Jephtha D. Howe of St Louis. In return for this information, Holmes promised

Hedgepeth $500 of the proceeds, a debt which, like all his others, he had no intention of paying.

By early August 1894 Holmes was out of jail and both he and Pitezel had arrived in Philadelphia where the fraud was to be set up. A run-down property at 1316 Callowhill Street was empty and available for a low rent, possibly because it backed on to the local morgue. There was a small shop and storeroom on the ground floor, with bedrooms above; here, under the name of B.F. Perry, Pitezel was to pose as a patent agent. It was sufficiently out of the way for him to keep a low profile, and he had enough knowledge of patents to convince a casual enquirer that he was genuine. Not that Pitezel was expecting to do any business in the short time it would take to carry out the fraud, and there was a convenient saloon nearby where he was planning to spend most of his time.

On 22 August a local carpenter, Eugene Smith, entered the shabby premises to speak to Mr Perry. Perry did not cut an especially impressive figure. He looked more like a manual labourer than a professional man, and there must have been a hint about him of drink taken. He looked older than his thirty-seven years, with watery eyes, a thin moustache and a wispy goatee beard. Smith explained that he had invented a saw-sharpening device and wondered if Perry could help him market his invention. Perry said he could and Smith returned home to get the model of his invention, which he bore excitedly back to the shop. He was less excited by the suggestion that he leave his model there, but eventually decided to trust Perry. Just as he was about to leave, another man entered the shop, a man who seemed displeased to see him there and anxious not to be noticed.

Smith saw Perry again on 30 August when he put up a rough counter for him in the shop, and was promised that matters were progressing well and there might be some news for him if he came round the following week. Pitezel obviously expected not to see Smith again, an expectation in which he was entirely correct. The last time Benjamin Pitezel was seen alive by anyone other than his murderer was on 1 September at the saloon.

On Monday 3 September Eugene Smith returned to the shop and finding it unlocked, he went in and waited for Mr Perry. The place seemed oddly deserted. Perry's collar, tie and vest were hanging on a hook, and his chair was standing at an angle in one corner. After a while, Smith departed, but he did not suspect anything was wrong until he returned the following morning and found everything exactly as he had left it. Smith decided to investigate and ascended the narrow stairs at the back of the shop. The front bedroom contained nothing but an unoccupied single bed, but in the back bedroom, from which an unpleasant stench was making itself known, there was the decomposing corpse of Mr Perry. Smith ran for the nearby police station returning with two officers who stopped on the way to summon a physician, Dr William Scott.

Scott made a careful examination of the body and its surroundings but a number of things struck him as very odd. At first sight death appeared to have been due to an explosion. The face of the corpse was swollen and black with putrefaction, but there was charring of the moustache and beard, and the front of the shirt was burned. Beside the body was a corncob pipe filled with tobacco, a match, and the pieces of a broken bottle. On the mantelpiece were a number of similar bottles labelled 'Cleaning solution – benzine chloroform and ammonia'. The police seemed satisfied that death was accidental, but Scott wasn't so sure. For one thing, the corpse seemed to have been laid out neatly, and neither the pipe nor the bottle looked as though they had been damaged in an explosion. The whole scene looked staged. Scott was also struck by the positioning of the body in the room, such that it would receive the maximum amount of sunlight on the face, hastening decay. If it had not been for Smith, the body might not have been found until it was unrecognisable.

The body was removed to the morgue, where Scott assisted the coroner's physician, William Mattern, in the autopsy. Death had been due to sudden cardiac failure. The lungs were congested and gave off a strong odour of chloroform, and there was liquid chloroform in the stomach. The state of the kidneys and stomach lining showed clearly that Perry had been an alcoholic, yet strangely enough there was no sign that he had drunk any alcohol recently. Mattern also noticed that the right arm, which had been resting against the chest, was burned on the upper surface but not on the part that lay against the body. The burning had been carried out after the arm had been placed on the chest; indeed, the nature of the burns showed that they had happened after death. The implication was clear – Perry had been murdered and someone had tried to conceal the cause of death and make it look like an accident. Mattern informed the inquest that Perry had died of chloroform poisoning, but the jury hedged its bets and found that death was due to 'congestion of the lungs caused by the inhalation of flame, or of chloroform or other poisonous drug',[6] which only went to show that they could hardly have understood the evidence.

It now remained for Holmes, assisted by Howe, to make a claim on the insurance policy, which involved first proving that Perry was none other than Benjamin Pitezel. Time had passed and it was necessary to exhume the corpse, which was now in a shocking state of decomposition, but Holmes, unperturbed, used a lancet to excise three identifying signs, a bruised nail, a scar on the leg and a warty growth on the neck. Pitezel's fifteen-year-old daughter Alice was obliged to identify her father by his teeth, the rest of his ruined face being mercifully hidden from her by a cloth. One of the party at the burial ground was Eugene Smith who, to Holmes's considerable embarrassment, recognised him as the man he had seen entering Perry's shop. By 24 September the insurance company, satisfied that death was accidental, paid up, and Holmes collected the money. Carrie Pitezel, who had been assured that her husband was still alive, received only $500.

It was Holmes's intention to dispose of the entire Pitezel family. Initially he managed to persuade Carrie, who was so distressed and confused by events that she hardly knew where to turn, that it would be best if he took charge of Alice and her younger sister and brother. Carrie never saw the three children alive again.

Justice was about to catch up with Holmes, however, in the unlikely shape of Marion Hedgepeth, who had read about the Perry case in the newspapers and was still waiting for his $500. On 9 October police headquarters received a letter from Hedgepeth, describing the entire scheme. Holmes was now a hunted man and with Pinkerton detectives on his trail it was only a matter of time before he was arrested. He was finally taken into custody on 16 November. It was not until then that Holmes's wife Georgiana discovered that not only did her husband have two other wives living, but another who was probably dead.

Holmes freely admitted the insurance fraud but insisted that Pitezel was still alive and the body had been supplied by a medical friend. The children, he said, were well and in safe hands. The case soon became a sensation. In the next few weeks evidence poured in of missing persons who had once been acquainted with Holmes. The brazen prisoner spun a variety of unlikely tales to explain the growing list of his victims. Eventually, when it was suggested that Pitezel's body should be exhumed a second time, he decided to make the best of a poor position and confessed that the body was indeed that of Benjamin Pitezel. He was not, however, about to admit murder.

The fraud, as Holmes said he had outlined it to Pitezel, was for his partner to feign death and be identified, then a body would be substituted for burial. Before he could obtain a corpse, however, Pitezel had taken matters into his own hands. At the end of August, according to Holmes, Pitezel had been drinking heavily and was suicidally despondent. On 2 September, Holmes had arrived at the shop and discovered a note written by his partner, which caused him to run up to the third-storey bedroom. There he found Pitezel cold and dead on the floor, with a towel over his face. Beside the body was a chair with a gallon bottle of chloroform, a four-foot rubber tube held in the bottle by a quill through a cork. The fumes in the room had been so strong that he had been obliged to leave the room and open a window. Once it was safe to re-enter he had dragged the body down to the second floor. Since the insurance policy would be void if the subject had committed suicide, Holmes said he had decided to fake an accident, so he smashed the bottle of cleaning fluid and set fire to the body.

There were a number of problems with this story. First of all, any evidence that it might have been true such as the suicide note, towel, tube and chloroform bottle had all supposedly been removed and destroyed by Holmes. It was also very hard to see how a gradual drip of chloroform could be obtained in the way Holmes described. The main difficulty was Holmes's description of the location of the death on the third floor. Pitezel's body had voided urine and faeces at the moment of death, and a stream of red liquid had issued from the mouth. There was absolutely no doubt that he had died exactly where he was found.

The bodies of the two Pitezel girls were finally discovered in July 1895, and with the certainty that Holmes was a murderer it was decided to examine the Castle in Chicago. There were sufficient human remains to suggest that the building had been used as a kind of 'murder factory'. The newspapers, which had until then characterised Holmes as a scoundrel and fraudster, now dubbed him an inhuman fiend. The hotel was all set to be opened to the public as a tourist attraction when on 19 August it mysteriously burned down.

At the end of August, after two months of searching, detective Frank Geyer finally found the sad remains of the Pitezel's young son, but when Holmes's trial opened in October 1895, he was charged only with the murder of Benjamin Pitezel. In a sensational start, the defendant discharged his attorneys and proceeded to conduct his own defence.

William Scott gave evidence that the cause of death was chloroform poisoning; moreover, he was sure that a man who had administered it to himself could not have arranged his body in the peaceful position in which it had been found.

Although Pitezel's stomach was inflamed it was an inflammation caused by chronic alcoholism, not the liquid chloroform found in it. Holmes, anxious to prove that he could not have chloroformed Pitezel while the man was drunk, elicited from Scott that apart from the chloroform nothing of any consequence was found in the stomach, not even a trace of alcohol.

It was Mattern's opinion that the chloroform had not irritated the stomach in the way he would have expected if it had been introduced there while Pitezel was alive, so he testified the extraordinary conclusion that the chloroform had been placed in the stomach after death. Mattern agreed on being questioned by Holmes that it could have got into the stomach by tube, but added that if it had been dripped into the mouth some of it would also have passed into the lungs, and no liquid chloroform had been found in the lungs.

Professor of toxicology Dr Henry Leffman did not think that chloroform could have been introduced by tube in the way that Holmes had described. He testified that if a man was lying on his back with chloroform dripping into his mouth, the direction of flow from mouth to stomach was uphill rather than down. He added that a liquid could not pass a dead oesophagus, as that would involve the act of swallowing, but agreed with Holmes that it was almost impossible to administer chloroform to a conscious adult male against his will.

It was felt that in general the medical evidence had gone against Holmes, and after it was done he reappointed his two attorneys. The most heart-rending moments of the trial came during the evidence of the sick and broken Carrie Pitezel, who identified fragments of her husband's clothing and told how after placing the three children in Holmes's charge, the next time she had seen them was in the morgue.

After the District Attorney's speech, which made a strong case, and exposed a great many of Holmes's lies, the defence would have seemed to have had a difficult task, but the young attorney made a number of valuable points. Why, he asked, would anyone put chloroform into a man's body after he was dead? Why try to fake a suicidal act when this would invalidate the insurance? Since Pitezel was not drunk when he died, how could Holmes have chloroformed him when the victim was a much taller muscular man, some 25 lb heavier? If Pitezel had been chloroformed in his sleep, why was he lying on the floor and not a bed?

Despite this excellent effort Holmes was found guilty of first-degree murder, and sentenced to death. Shortly afterwards he released a statement to the newspapers insisting that Pitezel had committed suicide. It was not until the following April that he finally confessed to the murder not only of Benjamin Pitezel but also twenty-six other people. Holmes was a practised and compulsive liar to the end. Two of his supposed victims were still alive, and another had died in an accident, while his description of Pitezel's murder directly contradicted the evidence he himself had been so anxious to elicit. Holmes claimed to have found his associate in a drunken stupor, bound him hand and foot to prevent him struggling, and burned him alive. On 6 May 1896, Holmes was hanged, taking with him the secret of how he had murdered Benjamin Pitezel.

Since Pitezel had not been drunk, and it was extremely unlikely that Holmes had overpowered him, the only other theory that seems to present itself was that Holmes succeeded against considerable odds in chloroforming Pitezel while he was asleep. One can reject the idea of Pitezel being bound, as there were no marks on the body suggestive of this. But if Holmes had indeed found Pitezel asleep, surely the murder would have taken place on the bed and not the floor? And how had he got chloroform down the throat of an unconscious man? The example of Edwin Bartlett suggests that if liquid chloroform is found in someone's stomach, then in the absence of any evidence to prove otherwise, it must have been consciously swallowed.

There is another scenario that has never been put forward. If the plan suggested to Pitezel was for him to feign death, and after identification for a body to be substituted, might he have submitted voluntarily to the inhalation of chloroform? Holmes was, after all, a medical man and could have persuaded Pitezel that he knew what he was doing, and that the procedure was without risk. The application could have started with Pitezel on the floor, the better to simulate an accidental death. What Holmes may not have known, since he had not practised medicine for a very long time, was that alcoholics take chloroform very badly. If Pitezel became agitated and was slow to go under, Holmes might have tipped chloroform down the throat of the partially stupefied man to speed matters up, then immediately afterwards stopped all pretence of a gradual administration, clapping the soaked towel against his victim's nose and mouth and holding it there till death supervened. The chloroform was not therefore introduced into Pitezel's stomach after death but very shortly before.

It would have been a messy struggle, with much chloroform spilt, and Holmes might have had to go out of the room for a few minutes and throw open a window to avoid being overcome by the fumes himself. On returning he found that the struggle, and callous pushing of the chloroform, had left telltale marks of murder. To conceal these Holmes attempted to burn the features then arranged the body in such a way that the face would decompose. This would make identification, which was essential to the fraud, more difficult, but he was confident that the distinguishing scar, bruise and wart would be sufficient. It only remains to speculate on why Holmes concocted a patently false story to avoid admitting how this murder had been carried out. Perhaps it was vanity. In common with many criminals of his type, Holmes liked to think he was cleverer than anyone else, and it would have been hard for him to admit he had been anything other than coolly efficient.

DEATH OF A MILLIONAIRE

Where chloroform and murder mix, the result is controversy. How was the poison administered? Was it even administered at all? One of the most celebrated murder cases of the early 1900s was the trial of Albert T. Patrick for the murder of the wealthy philanthropist William Marsh Rice.[7] Rice was born in 1816. He started his first business in Houston, Texas, and from humble beginnings built a substantial empire. Later, he and his wife spent much of their time in New Jersey and New York but maintained the business link with Houston. When the childless Rice decided to bestow his fortune on a charitable venture it was to be in Houston, the city that had made him. In 1891 a charter was drawn up for the William Rice Institute for the Advancement of Literature, Science and Art, and when Rice amended his will in 1896 the bulk of his estate was left to the Institute. There was, however, a complication. In April 1896 Rice and his wife had moved back to Houston hoping the warmer climate would help Mrs Rice's failing health. After her death in July, Rice returned to live in New York. When Mrs Rice's executor, Orren Holt, applied for probate it was found that only a few weeks before her death she had changed her will-without informing her husband. Claiming that she and her husband were residents of Texas, a community property state, she had thus felt able to bequeath half the Rice estate to her own relatives, considerably decreasing what Rice was expecting to leave to his cherished Institute. Naturally he contested the will, and a lengthy legal battle commenced. Holt hired a New York lawyer, Albert T. Patrick, and the legal proceedings dragged on for another four years.

Rice lived a quiet and lonely life, attended only by his young valet, Charles F. Jones. By 1900 he was eighty-four years of age, still in good health for his years and able to attend to business matters. The event that may have precipitated Rice's death occurred in September. A hurricane caused such severe damage to the plant of one of Rice's companies that the directors telegraphed Rice asking for immediate funds to carry out repairs. The sum required, $250,000, would effectively clear Rice's New York accounts of funds. Rice agreed to send the money, and sent an initial draft, but before he could part with any more, he was dead. Jones, who found the body, at once summoned a Dr Curry, who had been attending his employer, and also telephoned Patrick, who arrived carrying a letter from Rice authorising cremation. Curry obligingly certified death from natural causes, but Patrick seemed discomfited to discover that cremation could not take place for another twenty-four hours. In the meantime he agreed that the body could be embalmed. Patrick now attempted to secure the funds on Rice's bank accounts with cheques which appeared to have been signed by the old man the day before his death, but errors and doubtful signatures aroused suspicion, and the coroner sent the body for autopsy. This confirmed that all the organs of his body were normal apart from the lungs, which were extensively congested.

Another will now appeared, one that seemed to have been signed on 30 June 1900. Instead of leaving the bulk of his $7-million fortune to the educational charity, the main legatee was none other than Albert T. Patrick, whose main connection with Rice was that he was opposing him in a lengthy litigation. Both Patrick and Jones were duly arrested on suspicion of forgery. Jones, who was highly agitated, made a number of conflicting statements before attempting to commit suicide by cutting his throat. Once out of hospital he gave a lengthy statement, which remained substantially unchanged and formed the basis of his testimony at the trial.

According to Jones, he and Patrick had conspired to acquire the Rice estate. They had gone through the old man's private papers and discovered the original will, which left only small legacies to the Rice relatives. Their forgery cleverly increased the family legacies, and they retained the 1896 document, hoping that this would discourage the family from contesting the 1900 will. Letters were forged to suggest that Rice and Patrick had been in correspondence.

Even with these safeguards, Patrick was aware that he might have to resort to litigation to prove the will. Without adequate finances of his own, he counted on using the sums deposited in Rice's New York account, which he would secure with forged cheques.

None of these preparations are proof of murder. On the basis of this evidence alone, it could be suggested that the conspirators were content simply to wait until Rice died. On 3 August 1900, however, Patrick forged a letter from Rice authorising him to cremate his body. Such a procedure could only be carried out without autopsy if there was a certificate of death by natural causes, and to ensure that this would be forthcoming, Jones introduced Dr Curry, his own physician, to his employer. The stage was set for a rapid disposal of the body and any incriminating evidence.

The method of murder had, said Jones, actually been suggested by Rice himself. The old man had read an article about the dangers of chloroform, and discussed it with his valet.

Patrick sought Curry's advice, and the physician replied that if given in small quantities, which would only affect a man with a weak heart, the traces would be very slight. Jones had been giving his employer mercury pills, but these seemed to have improved rather than weakened his health, and in any case they would leave discernible evidence at autopsy. Early cremation was therefore vital.

Soon after the hurricane, and the planned emptying of the New York bank accounts, Jones tried to weaken Rice by giving him larger doses of mercury, but this was unsuccessful. When a messenger arrived on Saturday 22 September with a draft for Rice to sign Jones sent him away, saying that the old man was unwell and he should return on Monday. Curry arrived to examine his patient and found him weak but was confident he would recover his health. It really looked as though Rice would live to pay over the money on Monday.

Jones had already obtained some chloroform from his brother, and so, according to his evidence, on Sunday night, acting on Patrick's instructions, he soaked a sponge, put it in the apex of a towel rolled into a cone, placed it over his sleeping master's face, and left the room. Returning half an hour later, he found his master dead, destroyed the bottle, towel and sponge, and telephoned Patrick.

When the case finally came to trial, Albert T. Patrick stood alone in the dock charged with murder. Jones, the self-confessed murderer, had turned state's evidence against his accomplice in return for immunity from prosecution. Patrick's defence was that Jones was a liar, Rice had died a natural death, and the congestion of the lungs was caused by three pints of embalming fluid being pumped into the body. Patrick was found guilty and sentenced to death, but in 1906 Patrick's sentence was commuted to life imprisonment, and he was released in 1912.

It was not until 1904 that the legal difficulties concerning Rice's will were resolved. The Rice Institute opened its doors in 1912, and its distinguished academic record is all that its founder could have hoped for.

Martin L. Friedland in his detailed account of the case agrees with the defence. Jones had certainly not established a reputation for truthfulness, so why should his most recent story be the right one?

The first question to be addressed is whether Rice was murdered at all. On the face of it there is good, if circumstantial, evidence of murder. Patrick and Jones had an obvious motive, and the forged cremation letter showed intent to cause harm to Rice, while the giving of mercury, traces of which were found in the body, is evidence of actual attempts to do so. A crucial factor is the timing of the death. It is not impossible that Rice could have died of natural causes, although the autopsy gave no clue apart from the lung condition as to how this might have happened. However, that he should do so at the precise moment when it was most to the advantage of two men who wanted him dead is something of a coincidence.

The second question is how Rice died. Jones's brother testified that he had innocently supplied chloroform, and Jones's own testimony showed that he knew how it should be administered. A magazine with an article about chloroform was found in the apartment. It is impossible to be sure how the congestion of the lungs was caused. A demonstration carried out in 1906[8] showed that an injection of embalming fluid could reach and permeate the lungs, where its distinctive odour would be apparent. The original autopsy, however, had shown only that the lungs were congested with an excessive amount of blood, and no mention was made of any effect of the embalming. Post-mortem reports in deaths from chloroform where the lungs have been examined show that congestion with blood is a very frequent finding. Chloroform cannot therefore be ruled out as a cause of death.

One oddity in the case is Jones's claim that when he burned the towel and sponge it flared up as if oily. Chloroform is not flammable, and in any case after half an hour it would have evaporated. This seems to cast doubts on Jones's story, but he did mention that he had used a sponge which Rice had used to clean clothes with. It is possible therefore that there might have been some residue of a flammable cleaning fluid on the sponge.

Ultimately the question of whether Jones murdered Rice as described must rest on whether it is possible, as he claimed, to chloroform a sleeping man. Medical literature contains many accounts of the successful chloroforming of sleeping children, but whether it is possible to successfully chloroform a sleeping adult without the pungent aroma awakening the victim is a matter of some dispute. McIntyre reviewed the question in 1988,[9] and concluded that on the balance of available evidence it was possible, though difficult, and depended on the depth of natural slumber. He believed that in any individual case attention should be given to whether the account of what happened is credible. There are two points of importance in the Rice case – his age, which may have led to his requiring less anaesthetic than a man in his prime, and the fact that the chloroformed sponge was at the apex of a cone, and not applied to the nose directly, which would have made the vapour reaching him less pungent.

It is not proven that Rice died of chloroform as described by Jones, but it is not impossible.

THIRTEEN

THE ZEALOT OF HYDERABAD

> Have you ever known a dog faint? It is the rarest thing for a dog to have syncope. I have never had a dog that fainted, but my relatives are in the habit of fainting.
>
> *Dr Dudley Buxton*[1]

A prize-giving ceremony at the medical school at Hyderabad was not normally an occasion to set the world alight, even when, as in 1889, it was attended by the Duke and Duchess of Connaught. The presence of the royal guests did ensure, however, that the event would receive more than the usual attention from the press, and it must have been this that the Principal, Surgeon-Major Edward Lawrie, was counting on. The widely reported speech that he delivered was no dull congratulatory address but an open challenge to the London medical schools, arrogant, patronising, and impossible to ignore.

Lawrie announced that in the previous year, experiments carried out in Hyderabad had 'conclusively decided a question which had been in dispute ever since chloroform was first introduced'.[2] Chloroform, no matter how given, only affected the respiration, and was in no way dangerous to the heart. 'I have given chloroform as often, or oftener, than any man living, and have never had a fatal case,' he went on,[3] whereas in other places deaths constantly occurred, and would go on occurring until the London schools, which influenced the world, changed their principles, and ignored the heart, or 'confined themselves exclusively to the use of an anaesthetic like ether, which, with all its disadvantages, they knew how to manage'.[4]

As Lawrie threw down this gauntlet, doctors were looking back on their forty years' experience of anaesthesia, and assessing the lessons that had been learned. The consensus of opinion was that chloroform deaths were primarily due to stoppage of the heart. Even north of the Tweed, where Lister taught that only the patient's respiration should be watched, there was growing recognition that the pulse was ignored at one's peril. Those who distrusted chloroform were using nitrous oxide or ether, or embracing with relief a new wonder drug which they felt confident would have no complications – cocaine.

Lawrie was to stir this atmosphere of quiet debate into a frenzy. He was a man with a blazing passion for his subject, and an almost messianic determination to convert others to his ways, a man who knew beyond a shadow of a doubt that everyone else was wrong and he was right. He was born in Manchester, in 1846, the same year in which the Medical School of Hyderabad was founded, and qualified in medicine at Edinburgh, in 1867. A friend and fellow student was Thomas Lauder Brunton, although the careers of the two men were soon to diverge so widely that it seemed unlikely that they would ever meet again, let alone collaborate on a study which would cause a lasting storm in medical circles.

After abandoning a career as a ship's surgeon, due to persistent seasickness, Lawrie returned to Edinburgh where he acted as house surgeon to James Syme. Lawrie was a fervent admirer of Syme, and his belief in the essential correctness of Syme's teaching remained to the end of his life, unshaken by anything so embarrassing as contrary evidence. Syme had taught that chloroform only endangered the respiration and never the heart, and that was what Lawrie believed to the very last day of his life.

He was a man of immense energy, much loved by family and friends, who found him generous, witty and charming, and were sometimes dazzled by his impetuosity. Professionally, Lawrie sometimes showed the other side of that coin. He worked hard, and would tolerate nothing less in others. Dogmatic, determined and aggressively outspoken, he was utterly careless of whom he insulted in his insistence on establishing his perception of the truth. When he was sure of himself, as he was regarding chloroform, he spoke in absolutes, and he was not content, as so many doctors were, simply to express an opinion or publish a slim volume of advice. Lawrie needed to prove his case to the world.

Lawrie's readiness to leap to the defence of those he admired got him into hot water early in his career. In 1869 Joseph Lister had been experimenting with catgut ligatures steeped in carbolic solution. For the requisite degree of firmness the curing process took several months. Professor Spence of Edinburgh Royal Infirmary, holder of the most senior surgical chair in Scotland, decided to try them for an operation in which he was to tie the carotid artery. He asked for some ligatures and Lawrie gave him some that he had prepared only a few days before. According to Spence's account of the operation,[5] he had made careful use of antiseptics, but the patient died of unexpected complications three days later; when Spence examined the ligatures he found they had disintegrated. The new preparation was, he declared, 'by no means free of danger'. Lawrie, then only twenty-three, wrote to the *Lancet* asserting that Spence had not taken proper antiseptic precautions, thus suggesting that he was not only slipshod but a liar. The letter was published on 19 June,[6] Spence exploded in fury, and two days later, Lawrie was called before a meeting of the hospital managers and dismissed. Syme wrote a strong letter of protest, in which he described Lawrie as 'my excellent house-surgeon, than whom there has never been a better in my department of the hospital'.[7] Clearly, the admiration was mutual.

Lawrie joined the Indian Medical Service in 1872, and was to make rapid progress. While with a cavalry regiment in 1873, he had to perform a small operation on a lady and there was no one to give the anaesthetic, so he asked the colonel's wife to sit by the bed and give chloroform under his direction. She was so impressed that she wrote a letter of praise to her uncle, who just happened to be the Surgeon-General of the Indian Medical Service, and Lawrie was soon transferred to a better post in Calcutta. In 1885, as Surgeon-Major, Lawrie became Residency Surgeon to the State of Hyderabad, whose ruler, the young Nizam, Mir Mahboob Ali Khan, took an enthusiastic interest in the sciences, and gave every support to the work of the Afzulgunj Hospital. Lawrie was not isolated from European and American medical thought, but his stay in India had to some extent frozen him in time, cutting him off from the immediacy of key debate, and he was still Syme's man to the core, taking the words of the 1855 lecture as his infallible text. His reading of the current journals told him a dire tale of mortality under chloroform, deaths which he felt sure were preventable. He had personally chloroformed or supervised the chloroforming of many thousands of patients (he had not at this stage kept any statistics) without any deaths, and was therefore confident not only that chloroform could be perfectly safe, but that the secret of success was following Syme. Lawrie's method was simplicity itself. The inhaler was a canvas cone stiffened with thin pieces of cane, into the apex of which was placed a piece of cotton wool. The chloroform was poured on to the cotton wool and the cone held over the nose and mouth of the patient. The proceedings were managed and recorded by four students under Lawrie's careful observation. It was always the respiration and never the pulse that was looked to for signs of approaching danger.

Lawrie was aware that as a simple Indian doctor, an assertion of his superiority over the established leaders of European medicine might not be heeded. He started to keep statistics, and more importantly he persuaded the Nizam to fund a series of experiments. This study, carried out in 1888, came to be known as the First Hyderabad Chloroform Commission. In the nineteenth century animal experiments were carried out on whatever animal was most convenient to use. Often several different species were used in the same study. There was some appreciation that not all mammals reacted similarly to drugs, and a healthy distrust of the easy applicability of animal experiments to humans, but the finer details of the differences were a mystery, and the idea of selecting the most suitable animal to use for a specific procedure was in its infancy. Lawrie's study principally used pariah dogs, a half-wild breed similar to the dingo, which roamed the bazaars and were frequently rounded up and destroyed as pests. Altogether, 128 fully grown dogs had been subjected to experiments in which chloroform was administered in overdose. After the cessation of breathing the dog was revived by artificial respiration, and this procedure was repeated many times in each subject until the final test when it was allowed to die. To his great delight, the study proved what Lawrie had known all along, that death under chloroform always occurred by failure of the respiration.

Armed with his proof, Lawrie seized the opportunity to challenge the medical establishment in the presence of royalty.

The *Lancet* was not impressed with his experiments, of which very few details had been supplied, and pointed out that Lawrie's conclusions were at variance with the weight of European experience, which had demonstrated the depressant action of chloroform on the heart. Lawrie's response was, 'I hold that these views are wrong, and that there is no such thing as chloroform syncope.'[8] He suggested that if the *Lancet* could not accept his conclusions, it should urge the appointment of a commission. The *Lancet* declined to do so, demanding fuller details of the experiments, so Lawrie took matters into his own hands. He approached the Nizam, who agreed to provide £1,000 for the *Lancet* to send a representative to India to repeat the study.

On the face of it, it is hard to see why anyone had to travel anywhere. If Lawrie had simply provided a detailed report, then his experiments could have been repeated elsewhere, and the immutable truth of his assertions tested in other climates and with other animals. Instead, the *Lancet*, charmed by the generosity of the offer, accepted. Just one man was chosen, and that was Dr Thomas Lauder Brunton FRS, whose international reputation in pharmacology appeared to fit him admirably for the work. Brunton also represented the London point of view, in that he was of the firm belief that chloroform killed by stopping the heart. There were two possible disadvantages in the choice – Brunton lacked the necessary recent experience in the administration of anaesthetics, and he was also an old friend of Lawrie.

According to Lawrie he and the rest of the profession had agreed to 'stand or fall as regards the action of the chloroform on the heart by the results of the Commission's experiments. . . . The only reservation I made was that nothing the Commission could discover would persuade me that I could not give chloroform safely. '[9] It seems that Lawrie never seriously envisaged the possibility that he would be proved wrong.

Brunton sailed for India on 4 October 1889, and arrived in Hyderabad seventeen days later. It had been supposed that he would be the president of the commission, but Brunton at once relinquished that role to Lawrie, and was permitted only two days' rest before the work began. During his stay, Brunton was treated as a guest of the government of Hyderabad and a grand dinner was held in his honour, where he expressed the hope that the commission would finally find the answer that had been eluding science for so many years. In particular, the fact that instruments would be used to record the responses of the animals meant, he was sure, that the results would be free from bias, and the facts could not be challenged.

The experiments, carried out by Brunton, with materials and equipment donated by the government of Hyderabad, continued until 18 December, excluding only Sundays and holidays, work commencing at 7 each morning and ending at 5 p.m. Lawrie later claimed[10] that he had had no part in the direction of these experiments, but it is a little hard to believe that a man of his dynamism and convictions could have sat back without comment while others did the work on which his reputation relied. For reasons best known to himself, Brunton was unable to wait for a formal report to be issued before contacting the *Lancet*. Even before the work was completed, he sent a telegram.

> Four hundred and ninety dogs, horses, monkey, goats, cats and rabbits used. One hundred and twenty with manometer. All records photographed. Numerous observations on every individual animal. Results most instructive. Danger from chloroform is asphyxia or overdose; none whatever heart direct.[11]

This astounding message was met with stunned disbelief. Nothing could be done but await the final report which was made available in the following year.[12] It was studied minutely, debated and dissected, but more importantly, now that the world knew exactly what had been done, efforts could be made to check and replicate the commission's findings.

The majority of animals used were dogs, some healthy and some diseased. Importantly, the experiments were always carried out on animals which had already been anaesthetised. The main method of induction was to place the dog in a wooden box, and then gradually slip in pieces of blotting paper soaked in chloroform. There was a glass cover through which the animal could be observed, and once it fell over it was removed, and the experiment started. Chloroform was given by a variety of methods and continued until the animal died of overdose.

In every single case, respiration stopped before the heart. The critical experiments were those in which blood pressure recording apparatus had been used, adapted to show pulse-beats as well, and these yielded tracings on soot-blackened paper which were Lawrie's most triumphantly displayed evidence. To evaluate the dangers of shock, minor procedures had been carried out such as extraction of teeth, removal of nails or snipping of the skin of the anus, but there was no sign of syncope. The conclusion of the commission was that heart failure, if it occurred, was not a danger, but a positive safeguard, since it prevented further absorption and distribution of chloroform. Lawrie believed that the heart could only fail because respiration had already ceased, since one of his major articles of faith was that chloroform never affected the heart directly. But what of all the hundreds of deaths reported by others as having occurred with shocking suddenness? These, said the report confidently, had not been sudden at all, but had simply been missed because the chloroformist had allowed his attention to wander.

Those surgeons who had had the misfortune to lose a patient from unheralded cardiac arrest, the patient dying in seconds as though shot, must have wondered if their eyes deceived them on reading this passage. It could only have been written by someone who had never seen a human chloroform death. (The argument that Lawrie lacked experience as he had never had a death under chloroform was one which he was always to receive with some amusement.)

The report ended with a list of fourteen 'Practical Conclusions', which were effectively Lawrie's recommendations on how to administer chloroform. The only controversial statements were, first, that the administrator should be guided entirely by the respiration, and, second, that atropine was denounced as doing no good and possibly a great deal of harm. Years later Brunton was to say that the amount of work was so great it would have taken three years to make sense of all the tracings[13] yet the report was available a month after the work ceased. The full report was published at the Nizam's expense in 1891, and included the text of Syme's original lecture of 1855.[14] In the report, Lawrie admitted unblushingly that the Practical Conclusions 'were written before the commission had time to realise the full meaning of their experimental data or opportunity to put them to the test of clinical experience'.[15] One suspects that in Lawrie's mind they had been written before the commission had even begun its work.

The medical profession met the report with deep concern and scepticism. After all, if Lawrie was right, and chloroform was safe if given correctly, all those hundreds of deaths were due solely to carelessness. Matters were not assisted by Roger Williams, a surgical registrar, who tabulated the records of anaesthesia from St Bartholomew's Hospital for 1878–87 and concluded that the death rate from chloroform was 1 in 1,236, as compared with 1 in 4,860 from ether.[16]

The chief criticisms levelled at the Hyderabad Commission's conclusions were that human subjects could not be compared to the pariah dog, and that the results were in direct opposition to what had long been observed in clinical practice. A prominent sceptic was Dudley Buxton, administrator of anaesthetics at University College Hospital, who was rapidly emerging as one of the leading men in the field. The *Lancet*, anxious to compare clinical observations with laboratory results, asked Buxton to supervise a substantial study in which questionnaires were sent to prominent individuals and all hospitals with more than ten beds, asking for details of anaesthetic use, deaths and other dangerous cases, since 1847. While this was being done (and it took three years) matters moved on.

Although there were a few strident voices in Lawrie's favour, it must have become clear to him that his constant reiteration that the results put the whole matter beyond doubt were not having the desired effect. On June 1890, while in England, he asked W.H. Gaskell, lecturer in physiology at the University of Cambridge, to look over the tracings of the second Hyderabad Commission and report his conclusions, making any experimental investigation if required. Gaskell agreed, and the Nizam kindly provided £250 for the work. It was agreed that Lawrie would be supplied with a draft report, which he would then comment upon, before anything was published. Gaskell, working together with L.E. Shore, also of Cambridge, saw that the commission, which had declared that the fall in blood pressure during the administration of chloroform was harmless, had not tried to discover its causes. The Cambridge men, realising the importance of this point, devised an ingenious experiment, known as cross-circulation. The circulatory systems of two dogs were connected in such a way that if chloroform was given to one it reached all parts of its body, except the brain, supplying instead the brain of the other animal. This enabled the effects on the brain and the heart to be studied in isolation. Gaskell and Shore confirmed that chloroform did affect the heart, but more damningly, when they examined Lawrie's prized tracings, they saw that the curves did not support the conclusions of the commission at all, but just the opposite. Other physiologists were also at work, notably MacWilliam, who reported experiments on cats which showed that chloroform, unlike ether, resulted in dilation of the heart and consequent failure of the circulation.[17]

In 1891 Juillard,[18] one of the leading surgeons of the Geneva school, published statistics on more than 800,000 administrations of anaesthetics, which gave the death rate under chloroform as 1 in 3,258 and under ether as 1 in 14,987. He distinguished between primary syncope, which could occur during the first inhalations, and was sudden and dangerous, and secondary, which was slower, happened during deeper anaesthesia, and was characterised by a failure of the respiration. Lawrie, to whom it had not occurred and never did occur that his commission had only examined the second kind, triumphantly took the opportunity to compare Juillard's statistics with those of Roger Williams and his own clean record.[19]

Meanwhile, Gaskell and Shore, who had sent their report to Lawrie in August 1892, were waiting for his reply. They waited in vain. Lawrie's reaction was that since they disagreed with him, they must be wrong, and he set out to prove it. He did so by carrying out his own cross-circulation experiments in Hyderabad, and then publishing the results, claiming that they supported the commission, and quoting extracts of Gaskell and Shore's draft report without their permission. Gaskell and Shore, unamused at what they saw as a blatant attempt to suppress their investigation, went ahead and published.[20]

The work of the commission had also been received with great interest in the United States, where, by order of the Surgeon General's office, information was extracted from every American and European journal, and a report produced which concluded that ether was safer than chloroform and it was necessary to watch both the respiration and the heart.[21]

Nothing was ever going to shake Lawrie's utter conviction that he was right. He wrote repeatedly to the medical journals, accusing English doctors of incompetence and denouncing London teachings as dangerous. In 1892, he criticised a surgeon's attempts to resuscitate a patient by stimulating the heart. 'If the patient had only been left alone, and the safeguard action of the vagus had not been frustrated by the injection of ether, the stoppage of the heart would have saved his life,' he insisted.[22] When, in 1894, Gaskell admitted that the cross-circulation produced by his method might not have been 100 per cent effective,[23] this was Lawrie's chance to dismiss all the Cambridge experiments as a failure.

In 1893, the *Lancet* published a survey of the use of chloroform, which confirmed that no age group or nationality possessed an immunity to its effects, though there were more deaths among men than women.[24] The most popular method of administration was still the handkerchief. Returns for the USA showed that ether and chloroform were used with about equal frequency. In Germany and Switzerland, chloroform was used twice as much as ether, in Poland, the ACE mixture was favoured, but in all other countries chloroform was used almost exclusively. Where details of fatal cases were available, two-thirds were reported as due to cardiac failure, while in a significant proportion pulse and respiration had failed together, and in only one-fifth of the cases did it appear that respiration had failed first. The overall conclusion was that the safest anaesthetic for general surgery was ether; nitrous oxide should be used for minor surgery and dentistry, while 'chloroform, when given by a carefully trained person, is a comparatively safe body, but is not, in any case, wholly devoid of risk'.[25]

None of this had any effect on Lawrie's entrenched opinions. In March 1892, he had obtained funding from the Nizam for yet another study, this time carried out by H.A. Hare (who was later to give evidence at the trial of Albert T. Patrick) and E.Q. Thornton of Jefferson Medical College, Philadelphia. The results were sufficiently mixed for both sides of the question to take some comfort from them.[26] Hare and Thornton disagreed with the Hyderabad Commission's statement that chloroform was as safe as ether, observing that on the subject of ether the writers didn't know what they were talking about. They believed that the fall in blood pressure was harmful, unlike the commission, which thought it was a safeguard. The commission had stated that chloroform injected into the jugular vein did not paralyse the heart, whereas Hare and Thornton were able to demonstrate that it did, the commission's failure being due to poor experimental method. They even suggested that during administration it would do no harm to have someone watch the pulse. On the other hand they found, as in Hyderabad, that the respiration always failed first.

On 25 May 1894, Lawrie was in London, and attended a demonstration of the Hyderabad method by one of his assistants at the London Hospital, prior to which he had given a lecture in which he urged his listeners to abandon their firm convictions that chloroform acted directly upon the heart. The demonstration was successful enough, though it was felt that there was insufficient relaxation of the abdominal muscles, but after the years of clamorous promotion, many must have felt that they had not witnessed anything very extraordinary.[27]

Lawrie must have chosen to ignore the statistical work carried out by Frederic Hewitt, who was particularly concerned at the number of fatalities in dentistry, for which nitrous oxide had, by the 1890s, almost entirely replaced chloroform in London.[28] Collecting statistics for the fifteen years up to 1894 he found that chloroform was frequently used for dentistry in the rest of England and Wales and almost exclusively so in Scotland. Taking the relative populations into account he found that there were four times as many anaesthetic deaths in dentistry in England and Wales than there were in London, and eight times as many in Scotland. Since one could hardly suppose that Scottish dentists were eight times as careless as their London counterparts, the obvious conclusion was that the culprit was the anaesthetic.

By 1897, Lawrie was becoming increasingly sidelined. When Leonard Hill, lecturer in physiology at the London Hospital, delivered an address to the Society of Anaesthetists in London on the causes of chloroform syncope,[29] he referred to the Hyderabad Commission's 'ignorance of precise physiological methods' and the carelessness and incompetence of its experimenters. Like Juillard he distinguished between primary and secondary syncope, observing that the first was accompanied by paralytic dilation of the heart, while in the second the respiration was affected. Lawrie was hardly likely to let this go and there was an acrimonious exchange of letters in the *British Medical Journal*. Lawrie referred to Hill's views as 'exploded fallacies' and stated that 'deaths from chloroform are reported in the medical press by the dozen solely because the professional anaesthetists and certain physiologists refuse to be guided by the Commission's conclusions and still teach the false doctrine that chloroform produces direct cardiac syncope'.[30]

The practice of watching the pulse he denounced as 'frightfully dangerous'. Both Lawrie and Hill were at the Annual General Meeting of the British Medical Association (BMA) later that year, which wholeheartedly endorsed the work of Gaskell and Shore. Lawrie was quick to point out Gaskell's admission that full cross-circulation had not been achieved, and went so far as to read out a letter Gaskell had written to him admitting as much. The other delegates, notably Hill, were happy that the slight imperfection did not invalidate the results[31] but to Lawrie, this was his moment of triumph, and he later claimed it as a permanent and decisive victory.[32]

Even as he spoke, a new and more powerful movement was in the making. At the same meeting, Dr Augustus Waller, lecturer in physiology at St Mary's Hospital, London (later director of the physiological laboratory at the University of London and Dean of the Faculty of Science), read a paper stating categorically that most chloroform deaths were due to overdose and therefore avoidable, going so far as to suggest that they should be regarded as a criminal offence. Where Lawrie cited Syme, Waller cited Snow, and since Waller commanded greater respect than Lawrie, his work achieved far wider recognition.[33]

Lawrie could never see that the tone of his attacks almost guaranteed opposition to his views. 'The deaths under anaesthesia in England,' he wrote in 1898, 'represent an appalling picture of the incapacity of the medical profession as regards the administration of these drugs. This incapacity is altogether due to the absolute want of training of English students in the art of chloroform administration on Syme's principles, which have been established on a scientific basis by the Hyderabad Commission.'[34] This provoked a lengthy and bitter correspondence of which his detractors eventually wearied. Lawrie's confidence in his methods was unshaken even when in March 1899 a death occurred in Hyderabad. Lawrie was not present at the time, and the patient was a European, who struggled during administration. As was usual, the cap was removed to allow him to take some breaths and then replaced, but he died shortly afterwards. There had been 17,300 administrations in Hyderabad since Lawrie had commenced keeping statistics, an excellent record even without taking into account the years before 1889. It is unsurprising that Lawrie's confidence was such that he once got his granddaughter to give chloroform for him in an emergency operation when she was only eight years old.[35]

To examine the results of the Hyderabad Chloroform Commission critically it is worth looking for any cases which could, despite its conclusions, have been due to cardiac arrest. It is not necessary to look far. In nine cases, the animal undergoing the initial induction expired in the box before it was ready to be attached to the apparatus. Since the animal had died before the experiment proper commenced, its death was excluded from the experimental results, and it was assumed, without any supporting evidence, that death was due to failure of the respiration.

MacWilliam, who had also used animals chloroformed in an induction box, had a similar experience, but reported it very differently. Out of seventy experiments there had, he stated, been three instances of sudden cardiac collapse very similar to that seen in humans.[36] MacWilliam clearly demonstrated the direct weakening effect of chloroform on the heart, and believed that the blood-pressure readings on which the Hyderabad Commission had relied were 'entirely untrustworthy guides to the state of the heart under anaesthetics'.

Given Lawrie's splendid safety record with chloroform, it is tempting to think that he must after all have been in possession of some great truth, or extraordinary skill. He was not, however, the only person with a similar record; indeed, there were in general very few chloroform deaths in India. Many reasons were suggested, the healthier, predominantly vegetarian diet of the native population, more temperate habits, the looser clothing and greater circulation of fresh air, but one factor stood out – absence of fear. Dr Crawford of the Madras General Hospital stated that the Indians 'feel no alarm or uneasiness either about the issue of the anaesthesia or the operation. Habit, custom and climate all tend to lessen the native's fear of losing consciousness. He habitually takes opium and sees others go under its influence, and as he never hears of any deaths occurring under chloroform he has no reason to dread it.'[37]

W. Stanley Sykes, who was able to find records of only five chloroform deaths in India in twenty-five years, also pointed out that religious and cultural differences led to a calmer and more fatalistic outlook.[38] He reported a Dr J. Smyth of the Madras General Hospital commenting when he visited England after an absence of twelve years: 'What struck me chiefly was the look of terror on the faces of most of the patents as they prepared to submit themselves to the anaesthetic – nothing could be in greater contrast with all this than the happy anticipation of freedom from pain which, I may say, characterises our patients in the east.'[39]

In 1898 Arthur Neve of Kashmir submitted statistics on

chloroform deaths in India which showed a death-rate of about 1 in 26,000, a result he attributed to the climate.[40] Lawrie's record, while good, was not therefore exceptional.

CHLOROFORM IN THE NEW CENTURY

In 1901, Lawrie returned to practise in London, and published a book on chloroform administration which showed that time had done nothing to mellow his views. He continued to launch scathing attacks on English chloroformists, in terms ranging from patronising to plain insulting. Lawrie had nothing new to say, and in time his pronouncements came to be viewed as little more than an irritating noise. Lawrie felt that Lauder Brunton had failed to advocate the ideas of the commission as strongly as he would have wished, and in 1905 was unable to resist taking a dig at him by suggesting that chloroform was a far better treatment for angina that amyl nitrate.[41]

In 1900 the BMA published another study, which drew the unsurprising conclusion that chloroform was more dangerous than any other anaesthetic.[42] This meagre result was heavily criticised by Augustus Waller,[43] who shortly afterwards set up a committee chaired by himself, which included both Dudley Buxton and Vernon Harcourt FRS, reader in chemistry at Christ Church Oxford. The objective was to arrive at the best method of quantifying the amount of chloroform in the air and the body, and recommend an inhaler to control the dose. How long they expected to take in arriving at their conclusions is not known, but in the event this committee was to sit for nine years.

It was not until 1902, fifty-four years after the first chloroform death, that a study was conducted which focused attention on the dangerous period of induction, during which the majority of deaths occurred. Dr E.H. Embley, anaesthetist at the Melbourne Hospital, Australia, having observed a number of sudden deaths from cardiac arrest, conducted a study using dogs, and took the view that chloroform deaths were due to inhibition of the vagus nerve, which affected the action of the heart. He recommended that induction should never take place with more than 1 per cent of chloroform, and that concentrations above 2 per cent were potentially dangerous. The *British Medical Journal* had nothing but praise for Dr Embley, and confirmed the by now general belief that the Hyderabad Commission had failed to prove its main contention. (This drew the predictable furious retort from Lawrie.) The editor thought it 'curious' that these early deaths had not been investigated before – after all, as Embley's colleague Professor Martin had said of previous animal experiments, 'all the interesting things that occur in the box have been neglected'.[44]

Lawrie retired in 1909 to live in Hove, Sussex. Not that he was idle – he supervised the care of two mentally ill patients, one of whom was a relative of the Nizam, and continued to write passionately about the safety of chloroform. On the outbreak of the First World War he joined the staff of the Indian Hospital in Brighton. A contribution to the *British Medical Journal* in that year showed that his beliefs on the essential safety and methods of administration of chloroform were completely unchanged.[45]

He remained youthful and energetic almost to the end of his life, but died in August 1915 after a three-month battle with typhoid. The Nizam awarded his widow the not inconsiderable pension of £600 per year.

The value of Lawrie's work was that he forced the profession to re-examine the problem, and stimulated a great deal of debate and research. He did draw attention to the importance of maintaining a regular pattern of breathing, a valuable point when the amount of chloroform administered depended greatly on the respiration of the patient. It is also noticeable that in reports of chloroform deaths after 1889, doctors were taking greater care to record whether the respiration or the pulse ceased first. Not for nothing did Dudley Buxton refer to Lawrie as 'he who stirred the water'.[46] On the other hand, Lawrie also succeeded in clouding the issue by underestimating the dangers of chloroform and directing attention away from its effects on the heart. Those whose faith in chloroform had faltered had more reason to return to it, and those who remained faithful had all the more reason not to give it up. The object of the Hyderabad Chloroform Commission was to save lives, but the net result may have been to take them.

DELAYED CHLOROFORM POISONING

While debate raged about the effect of chloroform on the heart and the respiration, it gradually became apparent that there was another previously unsuspected way in which chloroform could kill. Quite possibly people had been dying in this way ever since chloroform was first administered, but since death usually took place hours or even days after the anaesthetic had been given the syndrome had never been recognised, much less recorded. A number of animal studies had already shown that in cases of prolonged administration of chloroform, there was evidence of fatty degeneration of the organs, but it was not until 1894 that the attention of the profession was firmly drawn to the fatal effects in human patients. The man responsible for highlighting the problem was Leonard Guthrie, house surgeon at Paddington Green Children's Hospital. In 1894 he published an article in the *Lancet*[47] describing ten cases, nine of which were fatal, all in young children, and all due to the delayed effects of chloroform.

The symptoms must have been truly distressing to watch, all the more so because of the helplessness of the medical staff to alleviate them, and the ages of the patients. Guthrie describes the condition as 'acute delirious mania' in which the children uttered shrill piercing screams. The eyes were dry, pupils dilated, the face could be either flushed or pale but often with a look of terror or anxiety. There were violent uncoordinated movements, and struggling, requiring careful attention lest dressings be torn off or fractured bones displaced. Violent, copious and persistent vomiting was an almost invariable symptom, the material resembling the dregs of beef tea. As the hours wore on, exhaustion set in, vomiting became less violent, the screams weaker, and a merciful unconsciousness supervened, leading to coma and death.

Guthrie's first such case had occurred in 1887, so these were not a frequent occurrence, nevertheless he observed the similarities and felt that chloroform was a possible factor. One remarkable feature in five of the patients was that on post-mortem the liver was found to be abnormally pale or fatty. Guthrie was not prepared to go so far as to suggest that the changes were solely due to chloroform, and suggested that the chloroform might have acted upon a pre-existing condition, though his opponents were not even prepared to go that far, and proposed a number of other causes. It took another ten years for the condition to be formally recognised and called 'delayed chloroform poisoning'.[48]

Even then Guthrie was still of the view that chloroform was only the last straw when there was pre-existing disease of the liver, though others were beginning to think that the anaesthetic might be wholly to blame, since it had been shown in animals that fatty degeneration of the liver could be produced in healthy organs after injections of chloroform.[49] By 1906 there were seventy known cases, many of them occurring in children with rickets, a condition caused by vitamin D deficiency, which then supplied a great deal of the surgical work in children's hospitals.[50] The connection between delayed chloroform poisoning and nutrition was not to be explored for some years.

In 1910 an observation suggested that chloroform was the primary cause of death.[51] An adult patient had died of delayed chloroform poisoning, and though, during surgery, her liver was observed to be normal, at post-mortem it was enlarged, bright yellow and fatty. In 1912 the American Medical Association Committee on Anaesthesia, concerned at the effects of chloroform on the liver, stated that the use of chloroform in major operations could no longer be justified, while in minor procedures safer agents were recommended.[52] The twentieth century saw chloroform fade from use – and then undergo an extraordinary rebirth.

FOURTEEN

FADE TO BLACK

> There are some of us who believe chloroform to be a most useful agent, which, if it could have been introduced today . . . would have excited the admiration of modern anaesthesiologists even more than it must have done with Simpson . . .
>
> *L.E. Morris, 1963*[1]

On 21 October 1972 a nineteen-year-old Wisconsin student was rushed to hospital, unconscious, his condition rapidly heading towards coma. The emergency revealed a recent craze for parties where a bottle of chloroform and a handkerchief were passed around the room for the participants' inhaling pleasure. Some, like the young man having his airways intubated in intensive care, also drank a small chloroform chaser after their beer. The patient was fortunate, and survived without permanent damage, and one can only hope that the chloroform parties ceased. Quite how they had started was never revealed.[2] In 1972 there was really no excuse not to know the dangers of chloroform, for by then the complex puzzle had been solved.

In the first decade of the twentieth century there was some confidence that the chloroform problem was approaching a conclusion. Nineteenth-century opinion on the subject had been polarised between the English and North American view of chloroform as a powerful paralysing influence on the heart and the Scottish and largely continental European view that it was easily controllable, and affected the respiration first. To some extent, this was still the position, but the experiments of the 1890s and 1900s had created another pair of opposing camps, the physiologists who studied anaesthesia under laboratory conditions, and the surgeons who observed the reactions of their patients. Some surgeons looked to the physiologists to solve the chloroform question, but others, like Frederic Hewitt, were convinced that for reasons not yet understood, chloroform anaesthesia was different in the laboratory and the operating theatre. There were two main schools of thought. Official opinion on chloroform deaths was led by Waller and Embley, who believed that deaths were always caused by accidental and therefore preventable overdose. The overwhelming evidence that most deaths occurred during induction, often with quite small quantities, had created a small undercurrent of opposition, which suggested that there was a particular danger in low doses.

In 1903 Waller unveiled what became known as 'Waller's chloroform balance', a device to measure and regulate the concentration of chloroform in air.[3] The difficulty with the simpler inhalers, such as Skinner's, was that the intake of chloroform depended on the patient's respiration, and Waller spent several years testing apparatus which could deliver the chloroform/air mixture at a constant fixed rate. Professor Dubois of Lyons had devised a mechanism which pumped the anaesthetic mixture into a face mask, and this was used by Waller in experiments in which he measured the chloroform in inspired and expired air when pumping the mixture into a bell jar containing a cat.[4] When the animals were deliberately overdosed, respiration ceased before the heart, but there was one case of early cardiac arrest.

Not that everyone liked the new inhalers. Vernon Harcourt's was often criticised for being too fragile and Dubois's for its weight. The low concentration they supplied also meant that it took longer to anaesthetise the patient. The two great advantages of chloroform – speed and portability – had therefore been lost.

Hewitt, who suspected there was a special danger in low doses, denounced apparatus such as the Dubois pump as cumbrous, complicated and likely to get out of order. He believed that it had been known how to avoid overdose since the days of Snow, Clover and Bert, but all these worthies had failed to explain deaths under light anaesthesia.[5]

Waller maintained that chloroform overdose could happen very quickly, even when it appeared that very little had been taken. He did not believe that low doses could be dangerous, commenting, 'we may as reasonably expect a man to be intoxicated because he has taken too little whisky, as to be killed because he has received too little chloroform'.[6]

When Waller's committee reported in 1910 it unsurprisingly recommended a maximum concentration of 2 per cent, and Vernon Harcourt's inhaler.[7] Unlike Lawrie and Lister, however, Waller admitted the existence of death by cardiac arrest, but was confident about the cause: 'a very high percentage vapour will cause sudden death – the death of the shot through the heart type'.[8]

The Vernon Harcourt inhaler enjoyed a brief period of popularity, but it never superseded the old favourites, the easily used, familiar and portable Skinner mask and Junker's apparatus, and their numerous modifications.

While the committee was being congratulated on its work, a dissenting voice was that of Alfred Goodman Levy, a former resident anaesthetist to Guy's Hospital, who was conducting research at University College Hospital Medical School. Levy conducted a series of studies on cats, which led him to a theory of the causes of chloroform deaths which was at once startling and attractive, for it seemed to explain everything. Having observed sudden death in lightly chloroformed cats, he had looked for, and found, evidence of ventricular fibrillation, a condition in which the heart is sent into a quivering flurry of rapid beats, which render it incapable of pumping blood.[9]

In subsequent experiments, he tried injecting the hormone adrenaline, which is a powerful cardiac stimulant, and in nearly every case this produced abrupt cardiac collapse. This did not happen under deep chloroform anaesthesia and neither did it happen with ether.[10]

Levy examined all available reports of chloroform deaths – there was no lack of these – and came to the conclusion that in every case where adequate details existed, contrary to the accepted view of the leaders of the profession, death was taking place under light anaesthesia and not by overdose.

By 1912 he was claiming that a similar effect happened in man,[11] as there had been a number of deaths after nasal operations, adrenaline being injected to open the airways and reduce secretions. Levy believed that chloroform created a state of irritability in the heart muscle, which diminished progressively as anaesthesia deepened. This in itself would not cause cardiac arrest – another factor had to be added. The other factor was adrenaline – and not only from injections, but the natural adrenaline produced by the body under conditions of stress, as might result, for example, from fear of an operation.[12]

By 1914, Levy was confident enough of his findings to read a paper to the annual meeting of the British Medical Association.[13] With a series of studies behind him, and the bit now firmly between his teeth he wrote:

> The theory of death by overdose has, in my opinion, been a most deplorable one for humanity; it is, I believe, the most unfortunate theory to which physiological science has ever set the impress of currency. I would urge upon those who still continue to lay exaggerated stress upon the risk of death by overdosage that they assume a grave public responsibility in regard to the perpetuation of chloroform fatalities.

There was no immediate acceptance of Levy's views, and in 1915 the *Lancet* warned against 'undue haste in accepting revolutionary views on chloroform methods'.[14]

Frustration was obviously setting in by 1917 when Levy wrote, 'I will not . . . waste words in an endeavour to elicit a response from the exponents of the overdose theory, for they appear to have wrapped themselves in the comforting mantle of dogma'.[15] The profession must have wondered if they had another Lawrie on their hands, but over the years his theories gained a wide acceptance.

It is impossible to judge what effect Levy's work had on the use of chloroform but it is interesting that chloroform's decline as an anaesthetic became noticeable around 1917.

THE FIRST WORLD WAR

The First World War saw the press calling for supplies of chloroform to be sent to the Front, and funds were started up to finance the sending of cases of chloroform to military hospitals. It was rumoured that shortages in France were so grave that operations had to be performed without any anaesthetic at all.[16] This may have been so in isolated areas, but the *British Medical Journal*'s special correspondent in northern France reported an abundance of supplies.[17] Cases of chloroform sent from England had actually been declined by French hospitals, which already had more than they could store, while chemists had plenty in stock, and could always get more from the manufacturer if needed.

Although press and public assumed that chloroform was the stuff to give the troops, and that without it there would be no anaesthesia at all, this was far from being the case, for while it still had a military role, it was no longer the anaesthetic of choice.[18] Sir Anthony Bowlby, consulting surgeon to the British armies in France, seemed to echo Sir John Hall when he stated:

> I believe that in [cases of shock or haemorrhage] it is safer to give no anaesthetic than to give chloroform, and ether is not much better . . . I am indeed inclined to believe that the success in primary amputations of Guthrie and his contemporaries would have been diminished if chloroform could have been given, and I am quite convinced that it should never be employed in such cases.[19]

Nitrous oxide was preferred but the supply was often limited, and it was saved for the most severe cases. While ether was primarily used, anaesthesia was induced with a chloroform/ether mixture as ether alone tended to cause some 'chestiness' and most of the men suffered from the effects of heavy cigarette smoking. Chloroform was also preferred to ether for induction in serious wounds where it was vital to avoid struggling.[20]

Lawrie's contribution to the war effort was the suggestion that the best and safest means of anaesthesia in the field was for casualties to administer chloroform to themselves using a Junker's inhaler in a manner very reminiscent of Dr Crombie's idea.[21]

BETWEEN THE WARS

As the century progressed, greater care and better equipment meant that the percentage of anaesthetic deaths in which chloroform was a factor decreased, but the increase in surgery overall meant that the largest number of chloroform deaths recorded in one year in England and Wales – 278 – occurred in 1933.[22] W. Stanley Sykes analysed chloroform deaths for the first 100 years, and found 24,278 in England and Wales alone.[23] Before 1911, any deaths under anaesthesia which were also related to strangulated hernia or cancer were recorded as due to the medical condition, and he thought that this may have led to an underestimate of 20 per cent. Given the relative populations of Europe and the United States, it would not be going too far to guess that in its first 100 years of use, chloroform was responsible for at least 100,000 deaths. The majority of these would probably have been avoided by the simple expedient of using a different anaesthetic.

Advances in anaesthesia kept chloroform in use for a few years longer – the development of more precise and controllable inhalers, the addition of oxygen, devices to maintain a free airway, and the use of intravenous anaesthetics such as thiopental sodium, for safer induction. In the 1930s chloroform remained popular for use in childbirth, and small capsules called brisettes, each containing 20 minims, were issued to midwives, no more than one per pain to be used for inhalation. The method was effectively identical to Snow's '*anaesthésie à la reine*' (sic).[24]

General practitioners still used the basic mask, and in 1936 some firm words were said to a Dr Choudhary after 27-year-old Mrs Marjorie Harris died at her home during a minor operation: 'The coroner said [chloroform] was now recognised to be a dangerous form of anaesthetic, and the doctor would probably be wise in dropping it. It was far better not to use an anaesthetic at all than to give chloroform.'[25]

THE SECOND WORLD WAR

At the outbreak of the Second World War, chloroform still had a place in the operating theatre and was considered to be the best anaesthetic for eye operations, providing what was called 'a quiet eye'.[26]

The old methods were still available in 1942, when this advice was given to the Australian military forces: 'Junker's apparatus and chloroform anaesthesia have fallen largely into desuetude. Occasion may arise, however, and especially in field units, when the apparatus may be turned to good account. Its use will be so familiar to the reader that a detailed description is scarcely required.'[27]

When, in 1943, medical student (later Professor) J.P. Payne was asked to give anaesthetics at Leith Hospital, he was handed a bottle of chloroform and a Schimmelbusch mask. Originally designed in 1890, this was similar to the old Skinner mask but with the added refinement of a gutter around the perimeter to prevent chloroform running on to the patient's face.

CHLOROFORM REBORN

Chloroform was destined to drift from use, with its unfortunate history of sudden death and a reputation for causing liver damage. In 1951 the *Lancet* commented: 'The feeling is widespread that to use chloroform when any other method is available borders on negligence. In spite of this many general practitioners find in chloroform sufficient good to make it their standby.'[28] As the twentieth century progressed, doctors were no longer expected to give patients general anaesthetics in their own homes, so the easy portability of a simple apparatus was no longer an issue.

In 1951, Ralph M. Waters, chair of the first academic department of anaesthesia in the United States, at the University of Wisconsin, initiated a series of studies which formed a milestone in twentieth-century appreciation of chloroform as an anaesthetic, for it provided the best picture to date of the effects of chloroform on the human patient.[29]

In one study, surgery was performed under chloroform on fifty-two patients, during which electrocardiograms were taken.[30] There were numerous examples of irregular heartbeat. One man held his breath for fifteen to thirty seconds during the induction, while chloroform continued to be dropped on to the mask, then suddenly took two very deep inspirations. He immediately went into cardiac arrest, but with prompt action he was revived. The recording showed not ventricular fibrillation, as Levy would have predicted, but an abrupt cessation of heartbeat brought on by sudden overdose. John Snow had been right all along.

Waters believed that by using accurate vaporisers to control concentration, and with care and close observation, chloroform could be used safely, and recommended that 'Chloroform does not deserve to be abandoned as a surgical anaesthetic'.[31]

We now understand the apparent paradoxes with which nineteenth-century doctors struggled. Where anaesthesia is slowly deepened, as in the studies carried out by Lawrie, and Thornton and Hare, respiration will gradually decline and will cease before the heart. This is what was often referred to as 'secondary syncope'. A sudden high concentration, caused by unsophisticated equipment, careless administration, or the deep inspirations of a nervous struggling patient, will stop the heart in an instant. This is the cardiac syncope that Lawrie denied existed.

As Snow realised, chloroform is far more potent than ether, and the safety margin between anaesthetic and fatal levels in the bloodstream is extremely narrow. In the early days of chloroform, lack of means to precisely monitor patients' vital signs meant that lethal doses could be given long before any danger was apparent. Chloroform does not irritate the airway, so even a tiny amount on a cloth can produce a high concentration, which can enter the lungs rapidly. There the blood becomes saturated with the vapour, which is quickly given up to the brain and heart. The irritant nature of ether is, curiously enough, a safety factor, since patients given it tend to cough, so initially smaller amounts reach the lungs. It is also much more soluble in blood than chloroform, and is therefore supplied to the brain and heart more slowly.

The heart versus respiration controversy is over – chloroform will affect both. It depresses the part of the brain that controls respiration and the rate and strength of heartbeat, but it also acts directly on the heart muscle, and its circulation, reducing its vital oxygen supply. It will also gradually paralyse the muscles which expand the chest wall during respiration.

Some patients are more at risk than others, for where induction takes longer than usual it is easier to give an overdose. For different physiological reasons this is most likely to happen with healthy muscular patients, those who are nervous and excitable, and alcoholics, three categories Victorian doctors would have immediately recognised. In India, where Lawrie and others had such a remarkable safety record, the calmer patients with temperate habits were far less at risk, and the warmer climate encouraged rapid evaporation of chloroform, which may have decreased the likelihood of overdose.[32]

It seems that Levy had been led astray by the fact that his work was done on cats, whose sympathetic nervous system is far more sensitive than that of humans. Nevertheless his observation that chloroform sensitises the heart to injections of adrenaline has been borne out by later work.[33]

Recent studies have also suggested that provided the patient is well nourished, and given additional oxygen, chloroform is no more likely to produce liver damage than other anaesthetics.[34] This knowledge has come too late, however, and understandably chloroform has been unable to earn back the trust of the medical profession, especially in the face of its modern rivals. Advances in chemistry in the 1950s resulted in the development of a new breed of non-inflammable anaesthetic ethers. Halothane was introduced in 1956, and others followed, with the arrival of desflurane and sevoflurane in the 1990s. But none are without risk, and while deaths under anaesthesia are rare, it is now accepted that the Victorian ideal of the perfect anaesthetic probably does not exist.

Where cost is a vital consideration, however, chloroform may still have a role, as it is far cheaper than its competitors. In 1981 Professor Payne[35] pointed out that there were many parts of the world where there was a need for a cheap, easily stored and portable anaesthetic: 'chloroform meets these criteria, particularly if used in the modern fashion using thiopentone [thiopental sodium] to induce anaesthesia, an established airway, and oxygen as a carrier gas'. Dr Harry Payne, former drug registration manager at Macfarlan Smith Ltd of Edinburgh, recalls that anaesthetic grade ether and chloroform were shipped to Africa until the early 1980s.[36]

In London, Professor Payne continued to use chloroform until his retirement in 1987, though by then his Schimmelbusch mask had long been superseded by the Chlorotec vaporiser, which supplied carefully calibrated percentages of chloroform mixed with oxygen.

CHLOROFORM AND THE MODERN CRIMINAL

There are still occasional cases where it is alleged that chloroform was used to facilitate crime. Professor Payne, who has been called as an expert witness in several criminal trials, believes that in order to give the jury a clear understanding of the medical issues involved, it is essential that both prosecution and defence should make full use of expert advice.

In 1994 he was a witness for the defence in a case where a 59-year-old doctor was accused of the abduction and rape of his seventeen-year-old receptionist. She stated that he had at first offered her a handkerchief to smell while he was driving his car, then, after stopping, held the cloth forcibly over her mouth and nose until she passed out. She awoke naked and tied to a bed, and the doctor was photographing her. Chloroform was again applied, and it was obvious when she awoke that intercourse had taken place. The question at issue was whether chloroform anaesthesia could have been induced as described by the victim, and maintained while the rape took place. The defence was that she was the doctor's girlfriend and had consented to everything that happened. The jury failed to reach a verdict, and the accused dismissed his counsel and engaged another who was less interested than his predecessor in the scientific evidence. At the retrial the accused was found guilty and imprisoned for ten years.

The occasional whiff of chloroform for aphrodisiac purposes is not unknown, but it is a hazardous business best avoided. In 1983 a 44-year-old industrial chemist stood trial for the murder of his mistress and for administering a noxious substance, namely chloroform. He admitted that they had used chloroform to enhance sexual pleasure, but stated that her death was an accident. The level of chloroform found in her blood was that normally associated with light anaesthesia, and it was probable she had died from inhalation of vomit. He was found guilty of manslaughter and given an eighteen-month suspended sentence.[37]

CURRENT USES

Many countries, following the example of the United States, now ban chloroform as an ingredient in drugs and cosmetics, and impose heavy restrictions on amounts permitted as manufacturing residues.[38]

United Kingdom legislation effectively confines the use of chloroform in medicines to that of a preservative.[39] In 2001 the *British Pharmacopoeia* still included chloroform spirit, chloroform water and tincture of chloroform and morphine, the twenty-first century version of chlorodyne. After 150 years of use there is still the occasional problem with solubility. In March 1998 two bottles of cough medicine at the Central Kowloon Health Centre were found to have a visible layer of chloroform at the bottom. It was found that the chloroform water had mistakenly been made with pure chloroform instead of chloroform diluted in alcohol, which is one-twentieth the concentration. Thirty-six patients had been issued with the medicine, and the Department of Health successfully contacted all but one.[40]

Chloroform is widely used in many commercial processes such as the manufacture of refrigerants and as a solvent for extracting natural substances; and it is an early part of the chain of production that eventually results in Teflon.

Chloroform has an invaluable place in the modern research laboratory, though reminders still need to be given about the dangers of decomposition. In 1999 it was noticed at the University of California, Los Angeles, that people working with three-year-old bottles of chloroform were suffering from chest pains, nausea and breathing difficulties. The safety data sheets had warned that phosgene would be generated from chloroform if it was exposed to heat and sunlight, but omitted to mention that it would also occur after prolonged storage.[41]

CHLOROFORM IS ALL AROUND US

We might be excused for thinking that outside the laboratory or factory we are unlikely to come into contact with chloroform, but it is all around us. The general population meets it in food, drinking water and air, and it is absorbed and distributed throughout the body, where it will be found in fat, blood, and internal organs, especially the liver, kidneys and lungs, as well as the nervous system. It has an especial liking for fat, where it will remain longest.

One of the main reasons for this is the chlorination of drinking water, which results in a number of by-products. Although chlorination has been used since the turn of the century, it was not until the 1970s that advances in analysis techniques confirmed that one of these by-products was chloroform.[42] This transfers to the atmosphere, where it may remain for several months before gradually breaking down. Not only tap water, but foodstuffs and drinks produced using it will all contain their little dose of chloroform. Most ingested chloroform is simply eliminated, by being exhaled.[43]

We can also absorb chloroform through the skin. Studies conducted in 1990[44] detected traces of chloroform in the breath of individuals who had showered for ten minutes in chlorinated water, where there had been none in the samples collected before showering.

Is there any reason for concern about the amount of chloroform in the environment? It is all a question of quantity.

There is a very considerable body of work on laboratory rodents which shows liver damage after exposure to chloroform, and this suggests that we should be careful to control long-term exposure; however the levels required for liver damage are very substantially greater than those we normally experience.[45]

While there is evidence that chloroform can cause cancer in laboratory animals, evaluations carried out since 1978 by the International Agency for Research on Cancer have found no direct evidence of a cancer risk for humans, and, in particular, have found no evidence of risk from chlorinated drinking water.[46] Overall, it is concluded that while chloroform may be carcinogenic in humans, the risk is low. On the other hand, the risks of not disinfecting the water supply are well known and very considerable. Where water is chlorinated, there are no longer the deadly epidemics of water-borne diseases such as cholera, dysentery and typhoid that ravaged nineteenth-century society. It is understandable therefore that controlled minute levels of chloroform in drinking water are generally considered to be acceptable. In the 1990s, scientists at the United States Environmental Protection Agency (EPA) recommended a maximum level of 300 parts per billion, below which it was considered that human exposure to chloroform posed little or no risk.

Chloroform's days at the centre of controversy are not entirely over, however, for in December 1998 the EPA ignored the conclusions of its scientists, and recommended a level of zero. In an extraordinary move, the EPA was taken to court by the Chlorine Chemistry Council and Chemistry Manufacturers Association in May 2000, and saw its decision overturned as 'arbitrary and capricious and in excess of statutory authority'.[47] Treated drinking water is normally expected to contain from 2 to 44 parts per billion, well below even the EPA scientists' recommendation.[48]

Chlorine is still the water disinfectant of choice, for its ease and effectiveness. Once used, it will destroy deadly infections throughout the water distribution system, all the way to the tap. One alternative is ozone, but that has its own by-products, and it breaks down quickly, so it will not ensure continued disinfection alone. Consumers concerned about the amount of chloroform in drinking water are advised to remove it by aerating the water in a blender. Boiling water will remove both chlorine and chloroform. Carbon filters are effective, but must be replaced regularly according to the manufacturers' instructions.

By far the greatest risks of high chloroform exposure are in the workplace, during the production or use of chloroform, or its indirect formation in industrial processes. Organisations such as the National Institute for Occupational Safety and Health in the USA and the Institution of Occupational Safety and Health in the UK exist to ensure that health and safety officers in the workplace have all the information they need to minimise those risks.

At the start of the twenty-first century chloroform's unique attributes put it at the forefront of science. A combination of chloroform and phenol is one of the most commonly used methods of extracting DNA and RNA from solutions of organic material, a procedure that has revolutionised genetic research and the detection of crime.

Recently chloroform has been used to achieve super-conductivity (conduction of electricity without resistance) with large carbon molecules.[49] At the University of California, a computer based on the laws of quantum mechanics has been constructed by passing radio-frequency pulses through a small amount of chloroform.[50] It seems that there is nothing chloroform cannot do – but we should always be aware of its dangers. As the great physiologist Flourens once said, it is both 'wonderful and terrible'.[51]

APPENDIX

THE CHEMISTRY OF CHLOROFORM

Chloroform

Formula: $CHCl_3$
Synonyms: Trichloromethane, trichloroform, freon 20, formyl trichloride, methane trichloride, methenyl trichloride, methyl trichloride, methenyl chloride, R 20 refrigerant.

The United Nations number (in the UK the Substance Identification number) is a four-figure code used to identify hazardous substances during transport. Chloroform is UN or SI number 1888.

CAS (Chemical Abstracts Service, the world's largest database of chemical information) Registry Number: 67-66-3.
Properties

1. Molecular Weight: 119.39
2. Boiling point: 143°F or 61.7°C
3. Specific gravity, where water = 1: 1.4832
4. Density of vapour, where air = 1: 4.12
5. Melting point: -82.3°F or -63.5 °C
6. Solubility in water: 1 ml in 200 ml water at 77°F or 25°C

The National Fire Protection Association has assigned a flammability rating to chloroform of zero.

Chloroform is classified as moderately toxic. Taken orally, the lethal dose for humans is between 0.5 and 5 grams per kilogram body weight. The average lethal dose is about one fluid ounce.

(Data from the United States Environmental Protection Agency Chemical Profile, 30 November 1987)

What happened in Samuel Guthrie's still

Since chloride of lime is a mixture, the equations given below are only a rationalisation of how chloroform was originally made.

1. $2C_2H_5OH + Ca(OCl)_2$ Æ $2CH_3CHO + CaCl_2 + 2H_2O$
2. $2CH_3CHO + 3Ca(OCl)_2$ Æ $2CCl_3CHO + 3Ca(OH)_2$
3. $2CCl_3CHO + Ca(OH)_2$ Æ $2CHCl_3 + (H\text{-}COO)_2Ca$

In words:

1. Alcohol (ethanol) and calcium hypochlorite give acetaldehyde, calcium chloride and water.
2. Acetaldehyde and calcium hypochlorite give chloral and calcium hydroxide.
3. Chloral and calcium hydroxide give chloroform and calcium formate.

The decomposition of chloroform

$2CHCl_3 + O_2$ Æ $2COCl_2 + 2HCl$

In words:

Chloroform and oxygen give phosgene and hydrochloric acid.

GLOSSARY

accoucheur a male obstetrician

ACE mixture an anaesthetic mixture composed of one part alcohol, two of chloroform and three of ether

adrenaline (epinephrine) a hormone secreted in response to stress; one of its effects is to stimulate the action of the heart

alkaloid a bitter nitrogenous substance found in plants. Many, such as morphine and quinine, have medicinal uses

amyl nitrate a drug used in the nineteenth century to ease angina pain as it dilates the blood vessels

analgesic an agent which relieves pain

aneurysm or aneurism a sac caused by dilation of part of the wall of an artery or vein, or in the heart

angina severe chest pain caused by lack of oxygen to the heart muscle

anodyne medication that relieves pain or discomfort

atonic quinsy an inflammation of the throat, with swelling of the tissues leading to danger of suffocation

atropine an alkaloid which stimulates the action of the heart

benzin (benzene) a volatile organic liquid obtained from distillation of coal-tar

carcinogen an agent which can provoke the formation of malignant tumours

cardiac syncope loss of consciousness due to an underlying disorder of the heart

carminative a medication that relieves flatulence

carotid artery a major artery in the neck, it carries blood from the heart to the brain

catalepsy a condition characterised by sustained immobility of posture

chirurgical surgical

chlorinated lime, or chloride of lime a white powder, usually a mixture of calcium chloride hypochlorite, calcium hypochlorite, and calcium chloride. Also known as bleaching powder

chloric ether originally the popular name of ethylene

dichloride, but it was soon applied to a solution of chloroform in alcohol

chloroform syncope cardiac arrest caused by action of chloroform on the heart

congelation production of local anaesthesia by applying a freezing mixture of ice and salt

delirium tremens syndrome suffered by alcoholics when alcohol is withdrawn, resulting in pain, tremors, confusion, and hallucinations

diffusive easily diffused through the system

drachm a liquid measure, one-eighth of an ounce, equivalent to 4 ml

Dutch liquid ethylene dichloride, so called because it was first made by Dutch chemists

electrocardiogram a record of the electrical activity of the heart

ergot a constrictor of the blood vessels used to control bleeding after childbirth by contracting the uterus

fumigant a substance which destroys pests or bacteria

galvanism therapeutic stimulation of nerves and muscles by a direct current of electricity produced by a chemical battery

gutta-percha a gum extracted from certain tropical trees which when heated and cooled retains it shape. Before plastics this had a wide variety of uses

grateful (of medicine) pleasing and comforting

halothane an anaesthetic gas introduced in the 1950s

henbane *Hyoscyamus niger*, a flowering plant, from which the alkaloids hyoscyamine, atropine and hyoscine are extracted. It has a long history of use as a sedative

hydrocephalus a build-up of fluid in the brain

hydrocyanic acid, or prussic acid a highly poisonous extract of certain fruit kernels

hypoxia lack of oxygen

hysteria a complex condition in which the patient loses emotional control, and suffers a wide variety of symptoms, including sensations of choking, convulsive movements, or motor paralysis

intercostal muscles the muscles between the ribs

lithotomy the operation of removal of a bladder stone

lying-in hospital a maternity hospital

mandragora *Mandragora officinarum*, or mandrake. Like henbane its extract supplies a mixture of alkaloids. The extract was much used in ancient times as an anodyne and soporific

manometer device for measuring pressure

medulla oblongata the part of the brain which regulates the action of the heart and respiration

neuralgia pain which extends along a nerve

oesophagus the gullet – the tube connecting the throat to the stomach

orchitis painful inflammation and swelling of the testicles

percussion powder powder so composed that it will ignite from a very slight percussion. Used to make gunpowder explode

pharmacopoeia an official published authority on drugs and medicines

phenol previously known as carbolic acid, used as an antiseptic in the nineteenth century. Among its other uses it plays a part in the extraction of DNA and RNA

phosgene carbonyl chloride, a toxic gas notorious for its use in chemical warfare, now with various industrial uses. Symptoms of exposure include coughing, choking, and nausea, which may be followed by an accumulation of fluid in the lungs leading to death

phthisis pulmonaris consumption of the tissues, tuberculosis

puerperal fever (childbed fever) infection of the genital tract after giving birth. Before the introduction of antibiotics this was often fatal

satyriasis persistent erection

specific gravity the density of a substance as compared with water, where water has a value of 1

strangulated hernia a hernia involving an entrapped loop of intestine

stertorous describes the deep snoring which accompanies some kinds of breathing

stricture narrowing, usually of a tube, due to scarring or growths

strychnine alkaloid drug – overdose leads to convulsions

sulphuric ether anaesthetic ether was so called in the nineteenth century because it was made by the action of sulphuric acid on alcohol

sympathetic nervous system the part of the nervous system which controls our reactions during an emergency, accelerating heartbeat, increasing blood sugar and perspiration, dilating arteries and slowing digestion

syncope sudden temporary loss of consciousness usually due to a reduction in blood supply to the brain

tetanus a disease caused by a spore which enters the body through wounds. Often fatal in the days before inoculation

thiopental sodium (sodium pentothal) a fast-acting barbiturate anaesthetic given by injection

tincture of capsicum alcoholic solution of an extract of the sweet pepper, used as an intestinal stimulant

typhus an infectious disease carried by fleas. Characterised by headaches, fever and skin eruptions

urethra the canal that carries urine from the bladder to the exterior

vagus nerve exiting the medulla, it has branches in the throat, gullet, lungs and heart. One of its many functions is to slow the heart rate

ventricles the muscular lower chambers of the heart which pump the blood to the body and the lungs

ventricular fibrillation very rapid uncontrolled beats of the ventricles during which the heart is unable to function

Vienna mixture anaesthetic mixture composed of 1 part chloroform to 6 or 8 of ether

Notes

Journal titles are given in their standard abbreviated form. A full list of journals and their abbreviations appears in the bibliography.

1 Give Me to Drink Mandragora

1. Alf. A.L.M. Velpeau, *New Elements of Operative Surgery*, ed. V. Mott MD (2 vols, New York, Wood, 1847), vol. 1, pp. 22–4
2. Genesis 3: 16
3. W.J. Bishop, *The Early History of Surgery* (London, R. Hale Ltd, 1964), p. 50
4. Ibid., p. 51
5. J.G. Beaney, *History and Progress of Surgery* (Melbourne, F.F. Baillière, 1877), p. 14
6. H.B. Gardner, *The History of Surgical Anaesthesia* (London, Baillière Tindall and Cox, 1896), p. 9
7. M. Grieve, *A Modern Herbal* (Harmondsworth, Penguin, 1977), p. 511
8. Bishop, *The Early History of Surgery*, p. 60
9. Shakespeare, *Antony and Cleopatra*, I, v, 6
10. Grieve, *A Modern Herbal*, p. 397
11. Ibid., p. 398
12. Gardner, *The History of Surgical Anaesthesia*, pp. 11–12
13. H.J. Bigelow, 'A History of the Discovery of Modern Anaesthesia', in *A Century of American Medicine* (Philadelphia, Henry C. Lee, 1876), p. 77
14. Bishop, *The Early History of Surgery*, pp. 95–6
15. J. Hennen, *Principles of Military Surgery* (Edinburgh, Archibald Constable and Co., 1820), p. 27
16. J.S. Dorsey, *Elements of Surgery* (2 vols, Philadelphia, Edward Parker & Kimber & Conrad, 1813), vol. 1, pp. 197–9
17. Gardner, *The History of Surgical Anaesthesia*, p. 15
18. Bishop, *The Early History of Surgery*, pp. 133–4
19. J. Duns, *Memoir of Sir James Young Simpson, Bart* (Edinburgh, Edmonston and Douglas, 1873), pp. 262–9
20. *Lancet* (1826), p. 647
21. H. Davy, *Researches, Chemical and Philosophical; Chiefly Concerning Nitrous Oxide* (London, J. Johnson, 1800), p. 556

22. Anon, 'Effects of Inhaling the Vapours of Sulphuric Ether', *Quart. J. Sc. Arts*, Miscellanea (art. V) 4 (1818), pp. 158–9
23. *Lancet* (1862:1), p. 366
24. H.M. Lyman, *Artificial Anaesthesia and Anaesthetics* (New York, William Wood and Co., 1881), p. 6
25. R. Fülöp-Miller, *Triumph over Pain* (New York, The Literary Guild of America Inc., 1938), p. 150
26. Duns, *Memoir*, pp. 220–1
27. *Pharm. J. Trans.*, VI, VIII (1847), p. 356
28. J. Shepherd, *Simpson and Syme of Edinburgh* (Edinburgh, E. & S. Livingstone, 1969), pp. 87–8

2 *Sweet Whiskey*

1. B. Silliman, 'Chemical Products Formed by Mr Guthrie', *Am. Jour. Sci.*, XXI, V (1831), p. 92
2. J. v. Liebig, 'Concerning the Discovery of Chloroform', *Liebig's Annalen*, 162 (1872), p. 161
3. V. Robinson, *Victory Over Pain* (London, Sigma Books, 1947), pp. 181–2
4. B. Silliman, *Elements of Chemistry, in the order of the lectures given in Yale College*, (2 vols, New Haven, H. Howe, 1830–1), pp. 19–20
5. B. Silliman, Appendix, *Am. Jour. Sci.*, Vol. XXI, V, p. 405
6. Silliman, *Elements of Chemistry*, p. 20
7. S. Guthrie, 'New Mode of Preparing a Spirituous Solution of Chloric Ether', *Am. Jour. Sci.*, Vol. XXI, I, Article VI, p. 65
8. Ibid., p. 64
9. B. Silliman, 'Remarks', *Am. Jour. Sci.*, Vol. XXI, I, Article VI, p. 65
10. Guthrie, 'New Mode of Preparing Chloric Ether', p. 65
11. J.R. Pawling, *Dr Samuel Guthrie, Discoverer of Chloroform* (Watertown, NY, Brewster Press, 1947), p. 45
12. Guthrie, 'New Mode of Preparing Chloric Ether', p. 65
13. B. Silliman, 'Remarks', p. 65
14. B. Silliman, 'Appendix', p. 408
15. See Appendix
16. O. Hubbard, 'Notes on the Discovery of Chloroform', *Trans. New York Acad. Sci.*, 7 (1892), p. 149
17. M.E. Soubeiran, 'Action of Chloride of Lime on Alcohol', *Ann. Chim. Phys.*, 48 (1831), p. 113
18. B. Silliman, 'Appendix', p. 406
19. Ibid., p. 407
20. J.B.A. Dumas, 'Chloroforme', *Ann. Chim. Phys.*, 56 (1834), pp. 113–20
21. Pawling, *Dr Samuel Guthrie*, pp. 51–2
22. Ibid., p. 57
23. G.B. Wood and F. Bache, *United States Dispensatory*

(Philadelphia, Grigg and Elliot, 1839)

24. J. Tomes, *Dental Physiology and Surgery* (London, John W. Parker, 1848), p. 349
25. J. Bell, 'Footnote', *Pharm. J. Trans.*, VI, VIII (1847), p. 357
26. *Lancet* (1871:1), p. 433
27. Duns, *Memoir*, p. 219
28. M.J.P. Flourens, 'Note Touchant l'Action de l'Ether sur les Centres Nerveux', *Compte Rendus Acad. Sci.*, 24 (Paris, 1847), pp. 340–4

3 *Adam's Rib*

1. W. Channing, *A Treatise on Etherisation in Childbirth* (Boston, William D. Ticknor and Co., 1848), p. 14
2. *Scotsman*, 27 October 1869, p. 7
3. Duns, *Memoir*, p. 252
4. Moreno, *Notes of Lectures of Sir James Y. Simpson, Archives of the Royal College of Physicians, Edinburgh* (1854), p. 75
5. Duns, *Memoir*, p. 253
6. 'Obituary', *Lancet* (1870:1), p. 715
7. Duns, *Memoir*, p. 81
8. Ibid., p. 93
9. Ibid., p. 128
10. Ibid., p. 123
11. Ibid., p. 111
12. Ibid., p. 334
13. 'Obituary', *BMJ* (1870:1), p. 507
14. D.W. Forrest, ed., *Letters of Dr John Brown* (London, Adam and Charles Black, 1907), LXX, p. 94
15. Duns, *Memoir*, p. 202
16. Ibid., p. 326
17. Ibid., p. 106
18. R.S. Atkinson, *James Simpson and Chloroform* (London, Priory Press, 1973), p. 35
19. *The Times*, 4 January 1847, p. 7
20. 'Editorial', *Pharm. J. Trans.* VI, VIII (1847), p. 350
21. *The Times*, 16 January 1847, p. 5
22. Duns, *Memoir*, p. 202
23. J. Pickford, 'On the Injurious Effects of the Inhalation of Ether', *Edin. Med. Surg. J.* (1847), p. 258
24. Duns, *Memoir*, p. 201
25. W.O. Priestley and H.R. Storer (eds) *The Obstetric Memoirs and Contributions of James Y. Simpson* (2 vols, Edinburgh, Adam and Charles Black, 1856), 2, pp. 739–44
26. Duns, *Memoir*, p. 231
27. H.L. Gordon, *Sir James Young Simpson and Chloroform* (London, T. Fisher Unwin, 1897), p. 108
28. J.Y. Simpson, 'On a New Anaesthetic Agent, More Efficient than Sulphuric Ether', *Lancet* (1847:2), p. 550
29. Editorial, 'The First Patient to Take Chloroform', *Brit. J. Dent. Sci.*, XLIV, 791, pp. 21–2
30. Simpson, 'On a New Anaesthetic Agent', p. 550
31. Ibid., p. 550
32. Ibid., p. 549
33. Duns, *Memoir*, p. 215

34. *Scotsman*, 27 November 1847, p. 3
35. Duns, *Memoir*, p. 224
36. Ibid., p. 216
37. *Lancet* (1847:2), p. 662
38. Minutes of meeting of Edinburgh Medico-Chirurgical Society, 15 December 1847, Edinburgh University Archives
39. R.M. Glover, *The Physiological and Medicinal Properties of Bromine and its Compounds . . .* (Edinburgh, J. Stark, 1842)
40. Duns, *Memoir*, p. 231
41. D. Waldie, *The True Story of the Introduction of Chloroform into Anaesthetics* (Edinburgh, Oliver and Boyd, 1870)
42. Duns, *Memoir*, p. 215
43. A.D. Farr, 'Religious Opposition to Obstetric Anaesthesia – a Myth?', *Ann. Sci.*, 40 (1983), pp. 159–77
44. Priestley and Storer, *Obstetric Memoirs*, 2, p. 622
45. J.Y. Simpson, *Answer to the Religious Objections Advanced Against the Employment of Anaesthetic Agents in Midwifery and Surgery* (Edinburgh, Sutherland and Knox, 1847), pp. 3–4
46. Letter of 27 December 1847, Simpson Archive, Royal College of Surgeons
47. *Lancet* (1848:1), p. 291
48. B. Brown, 'Chloroform Inhalation', *Boston Med. Surg. J.*, 37 (1847), p. 446
49. W.T.G. Morton, 'Results of Experiments in Boston with Chloroform', *Boston Med. Surg. J.*, 37, p. 447
50. 'Editorial', *Pharm. J. Trans.*, VII, VII (1847–8), p. 344
51. C.D. Meigs, *Obstetrics, the Science and the Art* (Philadelphia, Henry C. Lea, 1867), p. 375
52. *The Cambrian*, 11 Feb. 1848, p. 4
53. Lady Priestley, *The Story of a Lifetime* (London, Gilbert and Rivington, 1904), pp. 50–1
54. Duns, *Memoir*, p. 258
55. *Lancet*, (1848:1), pp. 291–2
56. Duns, *Memoir*, pp. 255–6
57. Ibid., pp. 258
58. *Lancet*, (1848:1), p. 184
59. U. v. Hintzenstern and W. Schwarz, 'Early Contributions from Erlangen to Theory and Practice of General Anaesthesia with Ether and Chloroform', *Anaesthesist*, 45(2) (1996), pp. 131–9
60. Robinson, *Victory over Pain*, pp. 232–3
61. *Boston Med. Surg. J.*, 38 (1848), p. 25
62. Priestley and Storer, *Obstetric Memoirs*, 2, p. 643
63. *The Letters of Charles Dickens*, Pilgrim Edition, Story G., Fielding K.J. (eds), 5: 486–7

4 *Under the influence*

1. Channing, *Etherisation in Childbirth*, pp.15–16

2. *The Cambrian*, 7 January 1848, p. 4
3. 'Eastern Dispensary', *Liverpool Chronicle*, 22 January 1848, p. 2
4. J.R. Hancorn, *Observations on Chloroform in Parturition* (London, Smith Elder and Co., 1848), p. 22
5. *Liverpool Chronicle*, 15 January 1848, p. 4
6. Moreno, 'Simpson's Lectures 1854', p. 153; Anon., 'Simpson's Lectures 1861–2', p. 101–2
7. Moreno, 'Simpson's Lectures 1854', pp. 151–2
8. T. Wakley, 'A Record of One Hundred Experiments on Animals with Ether and Chloroform', *Lancet* (1848:1), pp. 19–25
9. T. Adorno and M. Horkheimer, *The Dialectic of Enlightenment* (London, Allen Lane, 1973), p. 229
10. J. Pickford, 'On the Injurious Effects of the Inhalation of Ether', *Edin. Med. Surg. J.* (1847), p. 258
11. Priestley and Storer, *Obstetric Memoirs*, p. 534
12. R. Barnes, 'Observations on Dr Simpson's Anaesthetic Statistics', *Lancet* (1847:2)
13. Meigs, *Obstetrics*, p. 378
14. C.D. Meigs, *Females and their Diseases* (Philadelphia, Lea and Blanchard, 1848), p. 40
15. Priestley and Storer, *Obstetric Memoirs*, 2, p. 668
16. Duns, *Memoir*, p. 217
17. W.T. Smith, 'A Lecture on the Utility and Safety of the Inhalation of Ether in Obstetric Practice', *Lancet* (1847:1), p. 322
18. G.T. Gream, *Remarks on the Employment of Anaesthetic Agents in Midwifery* (London, John Churchill, 1848), p. 10
19. Ibid., p. 11
20. Priestley and Storer, *Obstetric Memoirs*, 2, p. 649
21. *Lancet* (1849:1), p. 100
22. Ibid.
23. 'Lecture at the Royal Institution', *Lancet* (1848:1), pp. 162–3
24. Ibid., p. 163
25. 'Chloroform and its Uses', *Lady's Newspaper*, 12 February 1848, p. 127
26. Duns, *Memoir*, p. 183
27. *Edin. Med. Surg. J.*, CLXXIV (1848), pp. 500–2
28. R.M. Glover, 'On the Post-mortem Appearances Produced by Poisoning with Chloroform Vapour and by Drowning', *Lancet* (1848:1), pp. 441–2
29. J. Abraham, 'On the Purification of Chloroform', *Pharm. J. Trans.*, X, I (1851), pp. 24–5
30. Moreno, 'Simpson's Lectures 1854', p. 126

5 *Her Majesty is a Model Patient*

1. Diary, 22 April 1853. *Lives and Letters. Queen Victoria in her*

Letters and Journals, ed. C. Hibbert (Harmondsworth, Penguin, 1985)

2. B.W. Richardson, 'The Life of John Snow', preface to J. Snow *On Chloroform and Other Anaesthetics* (London, John Churchill, 1858), p. xiv
3. *Lancet* (1858:2), p. 76
4. J. Miller, *Surgical Experience of Chloroform* (Edinburgh, Sutherland and Knox, 1848), p. 16
5. J. Snow, 'On the Administration of Chloroform during Parturition', *Assoc. Med. J.* (1853), p. 502
6. J. Snow, *On Chloroform and Other Anaesthetics* (London, John Churchill, 1858), p. 36
7. Richardson, 'The Life of John Snow', p. xxxv
8. *Lancet* (1849:1), pp. 209–10
9. Snow, *On Chloroform*, p. 201
10. *London Medical Gazette*, xlii (1848), p. 100
11. J.H. Bennet, 'On the Administration of Chloroform in Midwifery and as a Sedative of Uterine Pain Generally', *Lond. J. Med.*, XV (1850), p. 265
12. J.E. Pétrequin, *L'Ethérisation et la chirurgie Lyonnaise* (Lyons, 1869), pp. 1–5
13. *Bull. Soc. Chirurgie Paris*, 2 (1851–2), p. 336
14. *Lancet* (1849:2), p. 596
15. Snow, *On Chloroform*, p. 80
16. J. Gabb, 'Suggestions for the Employment of Ether and Chloroform in Conjunction', *Lancet* (1848:1), p. 521
17. *Lancet* (1848:1), p. 610
18. Ibid., p. 666
19. R.H. Ellis, ed., *The Casebooks of Dr John Snow* (London, Wellcome Institute for the History of Medicine, 1994), p. 259
20. Richardson, 'Life of John Snow', p. xxxvii
21. Ellis, *Casebooks of Dr Snow*, p. 271
22. *The Life of the Duke of Albany* (London, Crown Publishing Co. Ltd, 1884), p. 4
23. Editorial, *Lancet* (1853:1), p. 453
24. Ibid.
25. Richardson, *Life of John Snow*, p. xxxi
26. Ibid.
27. Ellis, *Casebooks of Dr Snow*, pp. 300–1
28. *Lancet* (1853:2), pp. 608–9
29. Ellis, *Casebooks of Dr Snow*, p. 471
30. H. Bolitho, ed., *Further letters of Queen Victoria, from the archives of the house of Brandenburg-Prussia*, tr. J. Pudney and Lord Sudley, (London, Thornton Butterworth, 1938), p. 105

6 *The Cure for All Ills*

1. *BMJ* (1862:1), p. 528
2. *Lancet* (1852:2), p. 90
3. Ibid., p. 6
4. *Lancet* (1850:1), p. 85
5. Edinburgh Medical-

Chirurgical Society, 'Minutes of meeting 7 June 1848', Edin. Univ. Archives Special Collection
6. H.W. Felter and J.U. Lloyd, *King's American Dispensatory* (Portland, Or., Eclectic Medical Publishing, 1898)
7. *BMJ* (1867:2), p. 280
8. *BMJ* (1855:1), p. 566
9. *Lancet* (1862:2), p. 579
10. *Times*, 'Sir James Crichton-Browne on "Food Fencing"', 18 September 1907, p. 6
11. *BMJ* (1851:1) p. 162
12. *Lancet* (1853:1), p. 535
13. *Lancet* (1848:1), p. 119
14. *Prov. Med. Surg. J.* (1848), p. 54
15. *Edin. Med. Surg. J.* (1848), p. 249
16. *Lancet* (1860:2), p. 117
17. *Lancet* (1866:1), p. 639
18. *The Times*, 28 January 1869, p. 10
19. *BMJ* (1864:2), p. 422
20. *Lancet* (1870:1), p. 445
21. *Lancet* (1848:1), p. 361
22. Snow, *On Chloroform*, pp. 52, 337
23. *Lancet* (1848:2), p. 39
24. *Prov. Med. Surg. J.* (1848), p. 353
25. *Lancet* (1849:1), p. 184
26. *Lancet* (1850:1), p. 136
27. *Lancet* (1850:2), p. 53
28. *Lancet* (1854:1), p. 393
29. Duns, *Memoir*, p. 217
30. *J. Brit. Pharm. Soc.*, XIII (1854), pp. 681–2
31. Priestley and Storer, *Obstetric Memoirs* (2), p. 765
32. *Lancet* (1857:2), p. 144
33. *Lancet* (1849:1), p. 564
34. *Lancet* (1853:2), p. 176
35. *Lancet* (1849:2), p. 122
36. *Lancet* (1867:2) p. 119
37. *The Times*, 15 June 1850, p. 4
38. *Lancet* (1855:2), p. 82
39. *Assoc. Med. J.* (1857), p. 226
40. *Lancet* (1854:2), p. 354
41. Ibid.
42. *Lancet* (1854:2), p. 513
43. *Lancet* (1858:2), p. 261
44. Moreno, 'Simpson's Lectures', p. 117
45. Ibid., p. 151–2; Anon., 'Simpson's Lectures', p. 67
46. *Ass. Med. J.* (1858), p. 718
47. Ibid., p. 252
48. *BMJ* (1868: 1), p. 323
49. W.G. Simpson, ed., *The Works of Sir James Y. Simpson* (Edinburgh, Adam and Charles Black, 1871), vol. II, p. 180
50. *Lancet* (1862:1), p. 518
51. *Lancet* (1863:1), p. 74
52. *Lancet* (1864:2), p. 49
53. Ibid., p. 71
54. *BMJ* (1866: 2), p. 217
55. Letter to Nunneley, 18 July 1869. Manuscript in Wellcome Collection
56. *The Times*, 5 April 1883
57. *Sheffield Daily Telegraph*, 15 February 1869, p. 3; 16 February 1869, p. 6
58. *Western Times*, 4 November 1864, p. 8
59. *Oxford University Herald*, 13 November 1869, p. 13
60. *Lancet* (1866:1), p. 24

7 Chloroform Goes to War

1. J.J. Cole, *Military Surgery, Being the Experience of Field Practice in India During the Years 1848 and 1849* (London, S. Highley & Sons, 1852, reprinted 1856), pp. 90–1
2. *Lancet* (1855:1), p. 349
3. 'Surgery at Vera Cruz', *Vera Cruz American Eagle*, cited in *Boston Med. Surg. J.*, 36 (1847), pp. 466–7
4. M.C. Gillett, *The Army Medical Department 1818–1865* (Washington, Center of Military History United States Army, 1987), p. 115
5. J.B. Porter, 'Surgery and Surgical Pathology: On the Effects of Anaesthetic Agents in Operations for Gunshot Wounds', *N. Y. J. Med. Coll. Sci.*, NS9 (1852), pp. 288–9
6. *Lancet* (1855:1), p. 196
7. A. Velpeau 'Gravity and Treatment of Gunshot Wounds', *Lancet* (1848:2), p. 5
8. C. Kidd, *On Aether and Chloroform as Anaesthetics, Being the Result of About 11,000 Administrations of These Agents, Personally Studied in the Hospitals of London, Paris, etc., During the Last Ten Years*, 2nd edn (London, Renshaw, 1858), pp.1–2
9. Cole, *Military Surgery*, p. 90
10. Ibid., p. 90
11. *Lancet* (1851:1), p. 96
12. J. Shepherd, *The Crimean Doctors* (2 vols, Liverpool, Liverpool University Press, 1991), 1, p. 59
13. G.J. Guthrie, *Commentaries on the Surgery of the War in Portugal, Spain, France and the Netherlands 1808–1815*, 5th edn (London, John Churchill, 1853), p. 585
14. Sir G. Ballingall, *Outlines of Military Surgery*, 4th edn (Edinburgh, Adam and Charles Black, 1852), pp. 378, 586
15. *Director General's Precis of Letters*, vol.1, p. 693
16. *The Times*, 14 October 1854, p. 7
17. *The Times*, 12 October 1854, p. 6
18. *The Times*, 12 October 1854, p. 9
19. *The Times*, 13 October 1854, p. 5
20. *Monthly J. Med. Sci.*, 19 (1854), pp. 475–6
21. *Med. Times Gaz.* (1854:2), pp. 506–8
22. E.M. Wrench, 'The Lessons of the Crimean War', *Lancet* (1899:2), p. 207
23. *The Times*, 23 March 1855, p. 8
24. *Lancet* (1855:1), p. 349
25. Ibid., p. 306
26. Letter from Dr Dawson to Sir James Simpson, 9 July 1857, Simpson Archive, RCS Edinburgh
27. G.P. Smith, 'On Military Practice in the East', *Lancet* (1855:1), pp. 647–8
28. *Med. Times Gaz.* (1854:2) pp. 664–5
29. G. Macleod, *Notes on Surgery of the War of the Crimea with*

Remarks on the Treatment of Gunshot Wounds (London, Churchill, 1858), pp. 131–6
30. G.J. Guthrie, *Commentaries on the Surgery of the War in Portugal, Spain, France and the Netherlands 1808–1815, with Additions relating to those in the Crimea in 1854–5*, 6th edn (London, John Churchill, 1855), p. 26, pp. 40–1
31. Ibid., p. 618
32. Ibid., p. 617
33. J. Snow, 'On the Employment of Chloroform in Surgical Operations', *Lancet* (1855:2), p. 361
34. Kidd, *On Aether and Chloroform*, pp. 22–3
35. MacLeod, *Notes on Surgery of the Crimea*, pp. 131–2
36. *Lancet* (1856:2), p. 79
37. M. Edwardes, *A Season In Hell* (London, Hamish Hamilton, 1973), p. 63
38. A. Case, *Day by Day at Lucknow* (London, Richard Bentley, 1858), p. 95
39. Ibid., p. 138
40. Ibid., p. 262
41. Ibid., p. 274
42. C. Kidd, *Chloroform and Substitutes for Relief in Pain* (London, Renshaw, 1872), pp. 121–2
43. United States Army, Surgeon-General's Office, *The Medical and Surgical History of the War of the Rebellion* (Washington, Government Printing Office, 1870–1888), 2(iii) p. 889
44. H.H. Cunningham, *Doctors in Grey, the Confederate Medical Service* (Louisiana, Louisiana State University Press, 1958), p. 226
45. *Lancet* (1861:1), p. 227
46. US Surgeon-General's Office, *Rebellion*, 2(iii), p. 889
47. M.S. Albin, 'The Use of Anesthetics During the Civil War, 1861–1865', *Pharm. Hist.*, 42 (2000), pp. 99–114
48. B.C. Smith, 'The Last Illness and Death of General Thomas Jonathan (Stonewall) Jackson', *Virginia Military Institute Alumni Review* (Summer 1975)
49. G.W. Adams, *Soldiers in Blue* (New York, Henry Schuman, 1952), p. 120
50. USA Surgeon-General's Office, *Rebellion*, 2(iii), pp. 888–9
51. Ibid., 1(i), p. 248
52. Ibid., 1(i), p. 254
53. Ibid., 2(iii), p. 889
54. Ibid., 1(i), p. 249
55. Ibid., 2(iii), pp. 890–4
56. Ibid., 2(iii), pp. 887–8
57. F. Haydon, 'A Proposed Gas Shell, 1862', *Mil. Aff.*, 2, 2 (1938), p. 54

8 *Murder, Mishap and Melancholy*

1. *BMJ* (1871:1), p. 97
2. *Scotsman*, 12 February 1848, p. 2
3. *Lancet* (1848:1), p. 218; *The Times*, 14 Feb 1848, p. 6

4. *BMJ* (1892:2), p. 827
5. *BMJ* (1860:1) p. 443, p. 484
6. *The Times*, 22 January 1848, p. 8
7. *London Medical Gazette*, NS, IX (1849), p. 478
8. BMJ (1849:2), p. 482
9. Editorial, 'The Administration of Chloroform by Gaslight', *BMJ* (1889:2), p. 184
10. 'Remarkable Misadventure with Chloroform', *Lancet* (1898:1), pp. 611–12
11. *Lancet* (1855:2), p. 367
12. *BMJ* (1884:2), p. 1201
13. *The Times*, 3 December 1875, p. 5
14. *Lancet* (1849:2), p. 541
15. *Lancet* (1860:1), p. 20
16. *Lancet* (1861:2), p. 6
17. *Lancet* (1853:2), p. 248
18. *The Times*, 22 February 1850, p. 5; J. Snow, *A letter to the Right Honourable Lord Campbell Lord Chief Justice of the Court of Queen's Bench, on the clause respecting the proposed prevention of offences bill* (London, John Churchill, 1851), pp. 9–11
19. *The Times*, 25 January 1850, p. 7; 1 February, p. 7; 9 February, p. 7; Snow, *Letter to Lord Campbell*, pp. 6–9
20. Snow, *Letter to Lord Campbell*, pp. 14–15
21. Ibid., p. 14
22. Ibid., p. 13
23. *Lancet* (1850:2), pp. 490–1; *Kendal Mercury and Northern Advertiser*, 19 October 1850, p. 2; Snow, *Letter to Lord Campbell*, pp. 12–13
24. Snow, *Letter to Lord Campbell*, pp. 11–12
25. *The Times*, 12 June 1857, p. 11
26. J.W.R. McIntyre, 'The Criminal Use of Chloroform Administered by Inhalation', *Med. Law*, 7 (1988), pp. 195–202
27. *Assoc. Med. J.* (1854), p. 692; Major A. Griffiths, *Mysteries of Police and Crime* (3 vols, London, Cassell, 1902), vol. 2, pp. 166–70; *The Times*, 31 July 1854, p. 12
28. *The Times*, 2 August 1854, p. 9
29. J. Hollander, 'Chloroform on the Orient Express', *Sunday Times*, 21 December 1975, p. 10
30. McIntyre, 'The Criminal Use of Chloroform', p. 198
31. *Lancet* (1851:2), p. 181
32. *Prov. Med. Surg. J.* (1851), p. 277
33. *Lancet* (1859:1), p. 400
34. R.J. Defalque and A.J. Wright, 'Robert Mortimer Glover (1816–59), Another Anaesthetic Tragedy', in B.R. Fink, L.E. Morris and C.R. Stephen, eds, *The History of Anaesthesia: Proceedings of the Third International Symposium* (Park Ridge, Ill., Wood Library – Museum of Anesthesiology, 1993), pp. 147–9
35. Records of Colney Hatch Asylum, London Metropolitan Archive
36. *Telegraph*, 13 April 1859, p. 6

37. *Lancet* (1859:1), p. 405
38. *BMJ* (1859:1), pp. 354–6
39. *Telegraph*, 13 April 1859, p. 6
40. *Lancet* (1852:1), pp. 360–1
41. *Lancet* (1853:1), p. 530
42. *Lancet* (1873:2), p. 60; *BMJ* (1873:2), pp. 92–4, 123–6
43. *Lancet* (1878:1), p. 816
44. *Lancet* (1888:2), p. 784
45. *BMJ* (1902:2), p. 562
46. *Manchester Guardian*, 27 October 1876, p. 6
47. *Runcorn Guardian*, 6 January 1877, p. 4; *Manchester Guardian*, 5 January 1877, p. 8; 6 January 1877, p. 8

9 Innocent Women

1. From letter written to Benjamin Waugh, 10 November 1885, quoted in B. Waugh, *W.T. Stead: A Life for the People* (London, H. Vickers, 1885), p. 6.
2. Duns, *Memoir*, p. 271
3. D.W. Buxton, *Anaesthetics and their Administration* (London, H.K. Lewis, 1888), p. 150
4. Editorial, 'Criminal Assault by a Dentist', *Med. Chron. Montreal*, 6 (1858), pp. 230–9
5. R. Ellmann, *Oscar Wilde* (Harmondsworth, Penguin, 1988), pp. 13–14; *The Times*, 19 December 1864, p. 6
6. *The Times*, 4 June 1870, p. 11
7. *The Times* 9 July 1867, p. 11; 13 July, p. 13
8. *BMJ* (1877:2), pp. 698, 708
9. *Birmingham Daily Post*, 10 November 1877, p. 8
10. *The Times*, 12 November 1877, p. 11
11. W.T. Stead, 'The Maiden Tribute of Modern Babylon', *Pall Mall Gazette*, 6 July 1885, pp. 1–6; 7 July 1885, pp. 1–6; 8 July 1885, pp. 1–5; 10 July 1885, pp. 1–7
12. *Pall Mall Gazette*, 9 July 1885, p. 6
13. 'Editorial', *Leeds Mercury*, 11 July 1885, p. 6
14. Letter from Havelock Ellis to Frederic Whyte, in F. Whyte, *The Life of W.T. Stead* (2 vols, London, Jonathan Cape, 1925), vol. 2, pp. 341–2
15. Whyte, *Life of W.T. Stead*, 2, p. 342
16. W.T. Stead, 'Bishop Frazer on the Social Evil', *Northern Echo*, 27 October, 1871
17. *The Times*, 24 October 1885, p. 4
18. W.T. Stead, *The Truth About the Armstrong Case and the Salvation Army, being the Editor of the Pall Mall Gazette's Statement in Full* (London, The Salvation Army Book Stores, 1885), p. 14
19. Stead, 'Maiden Tribute', 6 July 1885, p. 6
20. Ibid.
21. Ibid.
22. Ibid.
23. *Pall Mall Gazette*, 22 August 1885, p. 15
24. W.T. Stead, 'The Case of Eliza Armstrong', *Pall Mall Gazette*, 25 August 1885, p. 1

25. *The Times*, 3 September 1885, p. 10
26. *The Times*, 9 September 1885, p. 4
27. *The Times*, 28 September 1885, p. 13
28. Ibid.
29. *The Times*, 31 October 1885, p. 3
30. *The Times*, 3 November 1885, p. 3
31. *The Times*, 28 October 1885, p. 3
32. Ibid.; *Pall Mall Gazette*, 27 October 1885, p. 8
33. *Pall Mall Gazette*, 29 October 1885, p. 12
34. *The Times*, 9 November 1885, p. 3
35. *Lancet* (1885:2), p. 905
36. Ibid., pp. 972–3
37. Ibid., p. 973
38. *The Times*, 20 November 1885, p. 8
39. *Lancet* (1885:2), pp. 1209–10
40. Whyte, *Life of W.T. Stead*, 1, p.162
41. *Pall Mall Gazette*, 9 November 1885, p. 1

10 The Joy of Ether

1. *Lancet* (1874:2), p. 917
2. *BMJ* (1871:1), p. 452
3. Ibid., p. 480
4. Innominatus, 'Homicides by Chloroform', *Boston Med. Surg. J.*, NS5, 82–3 (1870), p. 113
5. *BMJ* (1870:2), p. 356
6. *Lancet* (1873:1), p. 897
7. Ibid., pp. 749, 846
8. J. Lister, *The Collected Papers of Joseph, Baron Lister*, Vol. 1(1), 'On Anaesthetics' (Henry Frowde OUP and Hodder and Stoughton, 1899) p. 143
9. Lister, *Collected Papers*, p. 153
10. Ibid., p. 149
11. *BMJ* (1871:1), p. 643
12. J. Lister, 'Chloroform Accidents', *BMJ* (1871:2), p. 118
13. A.S. Underwood, *Notes on Anaesthetics in Dental Surgery* (London, Claudius Ash and Sons, 1893), pp. 122–4
14. J. Clover, 'Chloroform Accidents', *Lancet* (1871:2), p. 33
15. Lister, 'Chloroform Accidents', p. 117
16. Ibid., p. 118
17. Ibid., pp. 118–19
18. Ibid., p. 119
19. *BMJ* (1871:2), p. 278
20. *BMJ* (1872:2), p. 575
21. Lister, *Collected Papers*, p. 153
22. *BMJ* (1871:2), p. 537
23. *BMJ* (1872:2), pp. 499–500
24. Ibid., p. 500
25. J. Morgan, *The Dangers of Chloroform and the Safety and Efficiency of Ether as an Agent in Securing the Avoidance of Pain in Surgical Operations* (London, Baillière Tindall and Cox, 1872), p. 21
26. *BMJ* (1872:2), p. 583
27. *BMJ* (1873:1), p. 234
28. 'Special Report on Anaesthetics and Anaesthesia', *Lancet* (1872:2), pp. 722–4

29. *BMJ* (1873:1), p. 194
30. *BMJ* (1879:1), p. 880
31. *The Times*, 22 July 1875, p. 8
32. *BMJ* (1876:1), p. 62
33. *BMJ* (1875:1), p. 627
34. Ibid., p. 760
35. *BMJ* (1875:2), p. 214
36. Ibid., p. 781
37. *BMJ* (1873:2), p. 11
38. *Med. Times Gaz.*, ii (1867), p. 590; vii (1868), p. 171
39. *BMJ* (1883:1), p. 917
40. J.M. Crombie, *The Induction of Sleep and Insensibility to Pain by the Self-administration of Anaesthetics* (London, J. and A. Churchill, 1873), p. 25
41. Ibid., p. 26
42. *BMJ* (1873:1), p. 672
43. *The Times*, 1 December 1883, p. 7; 4 December 1883, p. 10
44. *BMJ* (1876:1), p. 5
45. Ibid.
46. Ibid.
47. *BMJ* (1880:2), pp. 957–72
48. *Compte Rendus, Acad. Sci. Paris*, 96 (1883), pp. 1271–4
49. *BMJ* (1884:1), p. 281
50. F. Versmann, 'English Chloroform in Germany', *Pharm. J. Trans.*, S3, 2 (1871), pp. 63–4
51. Letter attributed to Dr Dott of Macfarlan Smith, private collection of Dr Harry Payne
52. *BMJ* (1882:1), p. 365
53. Ibid., p. 525
54. Rump, *Archiv. Pharm.*, October 1874; J. Regnauld, 'Production de l'oxychlorure de carbone dans le chloroforme', *J. Pharm. Chim.*, 5, 5, p. 504
55. *Lancet* (1882:1), p. 364; Lister, *Collected Papers*, pp. 160–1

11 The Crime of Adelaide Bartlett

1. Unless otherwise stated the facts in this case are taken from the full trial transcript, E. Beal, ed., *The Trial of Adelaide Bartlett for Murder, complete and revised report* (London, Stevens and Haynes, 1886); the handwritten notes of the magistrates court hearing held in the Public Record Office, Kew, ref CRIM1/23/7; official records of births marriages and deaths, and census returns
2. *South London Observer*; *Camberwell and Peckham Times*, 24 February 1886, p. 5
3. Y. Bridges, *Poison and Adelaide Bartlett* (London, Hutchinson, 1962)
4. *South London Observer; Poole and Bournemouth Herald*, 4 March 1886, p. 2
5. T.L. Nichols, *Esoteric Anthropology – The Mystery of Man* (London, Nichols, 1875)
6. J.B. Blake, 'Mary Gove Nichols, Prophetess of Health', *Proc. Amer. Phil. Soc.*, 106 (1962), pp. 216–34
7. *Lancet* (1886:1), pp. 968–70, 1017–18
8. P. Squire, *Companion to the latest edition of the British*

Pharmacopoeia, 12th edn (London, J. and A. Churchill, 1880), p. 99
9. Ibid.
10. Ibid.
11. Ibid.
12. Ibid., p. 100
13. *The Times*, 5 February 1886, p. 12
14. Author's experiments
15. F. Belman, 'Savior or Spy?', *Concord Online Monitor*, Monday 18 October 1999
16. K. Clarke, *The Pimlico Murder, the Strange Case of Adelaide Bartlett* (London, Souvenir, 1990)
17. 'A Chat with Miss Hibbard', *Nursing Record*, 2 December 1899, pp. 450–1
18. *Nursing Record*, 6 January 1900, p. 7
19. Archives of Bellevue Hospital, New York
20. R.G. Martin, *Lady Randolph Churchill, a Biography* (2 vols, London, Cardinal, 1874), vol. 2, p. 196
21. Mrs. G. Cornwallis-West, *The Reminiscences of Lady Randolph Churchill* (London, Edward Arnold, 1908), p. 330

12 The Sleep of Death

1. *New York Times*, 3 April 1901, p. 1
2. D. Robinson, *A History of the Dakota or Sioux Indians* (Aberdeen, South Dakota, News Printing Co., 1904), p. 227
3. *BMJ* (1870:1) p. 401
4. *BMJ* (1872:1), p. 347
5. The main sources for this case are H. Schechter, *Depraved* (New York, Pocket Books, 1996), and C. Bosell and L. Thompson, *The Girls in Nightmare House* (London, Gold Medal Books, 1959)
6. Schechter, *Depraved*, p. 116
7. The main sources for this case are E. Pearson, 'The Firm of Patrick and Jones', reprinted in *The Mammoth Book of Murder and Science* (London, Constable and Robinson, 2000), originally in *Five Murders* (The Crime Club New York, 1928) and M.L. Friedland, *The Death of Old Man Rice* (New York, New York University Press, 1994)
8. *Med. Leg. J.*, 24 (1906), pp. 329–30
9. McIntyre, 'The Criminal Use of Chloroform', pp. 197–8

13 The Zealot of Hyderabad

1. D. Buxton, 'An Address on the Practise of Anaesthesia in Oral Surgery: Its Dangers, Difficulties, and the Best Methods of Dealing with Them', *Journal of the British Dental Association*, XIII (1892), p. 615
2. *BMJ* (1889:1), p. 429
3. Ibid.
4. Ibid.
5. *Lancet* (1869:1), p. 772

6. Ibid., p. 888
7. Ibid.
8. E. Lawrie, 'The Hyderabad Chloroform Commission', *Lancet* (1889:1), p. 952
9. *Lancet* (1894:1), p. 1395
10. E. Lawrie, *Chloroform, a Manual for Students and Practitioners* (London, J. and A. Churchill, 1901), p. 10
11. *Lancet* (1889:2), p. 1183
12. *Lancet* (1890:1), pp. 149–59, 421–9, 486–510, 1140–2, 1369–88
13. *BMJ* (1915:2), pp. 350–1
14. E. Lawrie, T.L. Brunton, G. Bomford and R.D. Hakim, *Report of the Hyderabad Chloroform Commission* (Bombay, The Times of India Steam Press, 1891)
15. Ibid., p. 397
16. *Lancet* (1890:1), p. 349
17. *Lancet* (1890:2), p. 302
18. *BMJ* (1891:1), p. 920
19. Ibid., p. 1280
20. W.H. Gaskell and L.E. Shore, 'A Report on the Physiological Action of Chloroform, with a Criticism of the Second Hyderabad Chloroform Commission', *BMJ* (1893:1), p. 105
21. *BMJ* (1892:2), p. 936
22. *Lancet* (1892:2), p. 115
23. Lawrie, *Chloroform, a Manual*, p. 17
24. 'Report of *Lancet* Commission on Anaesthetics', *Lancet* (1893:1), pp. 629–38, 693–708, 761–76, 899–914, 971–6, 1111–18, 1236–40, 1479–98
25. *Lancet*, 'Commission on Anaesthetics', p. 1498
26. H.A. Hare and E.Q. Thornton, 'A study of the Influence of Chloroform upon the Respiration and Circulation', *Lancet* (1893:2), p. 996
27. *Lancet* (1894:1), pp. 1395–6
28. F. Hewitt, *An Inquiry Concerning the Safety and Sphere of Applicability of Chloroform in Dental Surgery* (London, J. Bale and Sons, 1895)
29. *BMJ* (1897:1), p. 786
30. *BMJ* (1897:2), p. 617
31. *BMJ* (1897:1), pp. 958–9
32. Lawrie, *Chloroform, a Manual*, p. 19
33. *BMJ* (1897:2), p. 1476
34. *Lancet* (1898:1), pp. 1681–2
35. W.S. Sykes, *Essays on the First 100 Years of Anaesthesia* (3 vols, London, Churchill Livingstone, 1982), vol. 3, p. 200
36. J. MacWilliam, 'Report on an Experimental Investigation of the Action of Chloroform and Ether', *BMJ* (1890:2), pp. 831, 890, 948
37. *BMJ* (1892:1), p. 296
38. Sykes, *Essays*, 3, p. 234
39. Ibid., p. 235
40. A. Neve, 'Chloroform in India', *BMJ* (1898:2), pp. 1418–20
41. *Lancet* (1905:1), p. 922
42. *BMJ* (1901:1), p. 163
43. Ibid., pp. 447–8

44. *BMJ* (1902:1), pp. 975–6
45. *BMJ* (1914:1), p. 623
46. *Lancet* (1915:2), p. 676
47. L.G. Guthrie, 'On Some Fatal After-effects of Chloroform on Children', *Lancet* (1894:1), pp. 193–4
48. *Lancet* (1904:1), p. 1657
49. *Lancet* (1905:2), pp. 437–40
50. E.D. Telford and J.L. Falconer, 'Delayed Chloroform Poisoning', *Lancet* (1906:2), pp. 1341–3
51. E.D. Telford, 'Some Notes on "Delayed Chloroform Poisoning"' *Lancet* (1910:2), pp. 1269–70
52. Y. Henderson, T.S. Cullen, E.D. Martin, T.W. Huntington, F.T. Murphy, 'Report of Committee on Anesthesia', *JAMA*, 58 (1912)

14. Fade to Black

1. L.E. Morris, 'Chloroform', *Clin. Anesth.*, 1 (1963), p. 24
2. W.W. Storms, 'Chloroform Parties', *JAMA*, 225(2) (1973), p. 160
3. A.D. Waller and V. Geets, 'The Rapid Estimation of the Quantity of Chloroform Vapour in Mixtures of Chloroform Vapour and Air', *BMJ* (1903:1), pp. 1421–5
4. A.D. Waller, 'The Administration of Chloroform to Man and the Higher Animals', *Lancet* (1903:1), pp. 1481–6
5. *Lancet* (1904:2), pp. 1496–9
6. *Lancet* (1904:2), p. 978
7. *BMJ*, 1910 supp, pp. 47–72
8. *BMJ* (1910:2), p. 752
9. A.G. Levy, 'Sudden Death under Chloroform', *J. Physiol*, 42 (1911), pp. iii–vii
10. Ibid., p. vii
11. A.G. Levy, 'A Cardiac Reaction to Adrenaline in Chloroformed Subjects', *Lancet* (1912:2), p. 524
12. A.G. Levy, *Chloroform Anaesthesia* (London, John Bale Sons and Danielsson, 1922), p. 136
13. A.G. Levy, 'Ventricular Fibrillation, the Cause of Death under Chloroform', *BMJ* (1914:2), pp. 502–3
14. *Lancet* (1915:2), p. 296
15. *BMJ* (1917:1), p. 65
16. *Lancet* (1914:2), pp. 1126, 1278
17. 'From a Special Correspondent in Northern France', *BMJ* (1914:2), pp. 1079–80
18. H.C. Bazett, 'On Shock and Haemorrhage', Chapter 13 in *A Manual of War Surgery*, ed. S. Barling and J.T. Morrison (London, Frowde and Hodder and Stoughton, 1919), pp. 397–412
19. A. Bowlby, *The Hunterian Oration on British Military Surgery in the Time of Hunter and in the Great War* (London, Adlard and Son and West Newman, 1919)
20. A.S. Daly, 'Anaesthetics',

Chapter 15 in Barling, pp. 429–35
21. *BMJ* (1914:2), p. 690
22. Sykes, *Essays*, 2, p. 36
23. Sykes, *Essays*, 2, p. 39
24. *Brit. J. Anesth.*, XI (1933–4), p. 29
25. *The Times*, 6 October 1936, p. 8
26. J.P. Payne, 'Anaesthetic Training in Wartime Britain', *World Anaesthesia* (1999) 3, 1, article 3
27. G. Kaye, *Manual of Army Anaesthetic Apparatus* (Melbourne, Australian Military Forces, 1942), p. 50
28. *Lancet* (1951:2), p. 57
29. R.M. Waters, ed., *Chloroform, a Study after 100 Years* (Madison, University of Wisconsin Press, 1951)
30. O.S. Orth, R.R. Liebenow and R.T. Capps, 'The Effect of Chloroform on the Cardio-vascular System', in *Chloroform, a Study*, pp. 40–75
31. Waters, *Chloroform, a Study*, p. 124
32. The author is indebted to Dr Ray Defalque for his advice on the effects of chloroform anaesthesia
33. W.J. Meek, 'Cardiac Automaticity and Response to Blood Pressure Raising Agents during Inhalation Anaesthesia', *Physiol. Reviews*, 21 (1941), pp. 324–56
34. W.N. Rollason, 'Chloroform, Halothane and Hepatotoxicity', *Proc. Roy. Soc. Med.*, 57 (1964), p. 307; S.A. Oduntan, 'Chloroform Anaesthesia – a Clinical Comparison of Chloroform and Halothane Administered from Precision Vaporisers', *Anaesthesia*, 23 (1968), p. 552
35. J.P. Payne, 'Chloroform in Clinical Anaesthesia', *Brit. J. Anesth.* 53 (1981), p. 11S
36. Personal communication
37. J.P. Payne, 'The Criminal Use of Chloroform', *Anaesthesia*, 53 (1998), pp. 685–90
38. United States Food and Drug Administration, *Chloroform as an Ingredient of Human Drug and Cosmetic Products*, Fed. Reg. 41:26842–5 (1976); United States Food and Drug Administration, *Guidance for Industry: Q3C Impurities: Residual Solvents* (1997)
39. The Medicines (Chloroform Prohibition) Order 1979 (SI 1979 No. 382, amended by SI 1980/263)
40. Panel on Health Services (papers), 'Dispensing Error at Central Kowloon Health Centre' (Information Note, March 1998, Kowloon)
41. *Environmental Health and Safety Newsletter* (Medical College of Georgia, Fall 1999)
42. P.C. Singer, ed., *Formation and Control of Disinfection By-products in Drinking Water* (Denver, American Water Works Association, 1999), pp. 2–3

43. J. Fry, R. Taylor, and D.E. Hathaway, 'Pulmonary Elimination of Chloroform and its Metabolite in Man', *Arch. Int. Pharmacodyn. Ther.*, 196 (1972), pp. 98–111
44. W.K. Jo, C.P. Weisel, and P.J. Lioy, 'Routes of Chloroform Exposure and Body Burden from Showering with Chlorinated Tap Water', *Risk Anal.* 10 (1990a), pp. 575–80; Jo *et al.*, 'Chloroform Exposure and the Health Risk Associated with Multiple Uses of Chlorinated Tap Water', *Risk Anal.* 10 (1990b), pp. 581–5
45. Agency for Toxic Substances and Disease Registry (ATSDR), 'Toxicological Profile for Chloroform' (Atlanta, GA, Public Health Service, US Department of Health and Human Services, 1997); U. Lahl, K. Bätjer, J. v Düszeln, B. Gabel, B. Stachel, and W. Thiemann, 'Distribution and Balance of Volatile Halogenated Hydrocarbons in the Water and Air of Covered Swimming Pools using Chlorine for Water Disinfection', *Water Res.* 15 (1981a), pp. 803–14; H.A. Bomski, A. Sobdewska and A. Strakowski, 'Toxic Damage of the Liver by Chloroform in Chemical Industry Workers', *Int. Arch. Gewerbepathol. Gewerbehyg.*, 24 (1967) pp. 127–34; W.H. Phoon, K.T. Goh, L.T. Lee, K.T. Tan, and S.F. Kwok, 'Toxic Jaundice from Occupational Exposure to Chloroform', *Med. J. Malays.*, 38 (1983), pp. 31–4
46. 'Chloroform', *International Agency for Research on Cancer, Summary and Evaluation*, vol. 1 (1972), vol. 20 (1979), supp. 7 (1987)
47. B.R. Cohen, 'Court Rejects EPA Chloroform Rule', *Environment and Climate News*, June 2000
48. Agency for Toxic Substances and Disease Registry, 'Toxicological Profile for Chloroform' (United States Public Health Service, August 1995 update)
49. 'The Straight Dope on Superconductivity', *Science*, 293 (2001), p. 2345
50. N. Gershenfeld and I.L. Chuang, 'Quantum Computing with Molecules', *Sci. Am.*, (June 1998)
51. Alf. A.L.M Velpeau, and M.J.P Flourens, 'Communications relatives au chloroforme', *Séance de l'Académie des sciences du 13 Décembre 1847, Union Med.* 1 (1847), p. 631

Bibliography

Adams, G.W., *Soldiers in Blue*, New York, Henry Schuman, 1952

Agency for Toxic Substances and Disease Registry (ATSDR), *Toxicological Profile for Chloroform*, Atlanta, GA, Public Health Service, US Department of Health and Human Services, 1997

Alphandery, M.-F., *Dictionnaire des Inventeurs Français*, Paris, Collection Seghers,1962

American Water Works Association, *Fact sheet, Trihalomethanes (THMs)*, 2002

Anonymous, *The Life of the Duke of Albany*, London, Crown Publishing Company, 1884

——, *The Life of Mr W.T. Stead*, London, John Kensit, 1886

——, *Notes of Lectures of Sir James Y. Simpson* (1861–2), Archives of the Royal College of Physicians, Edinburgh

Atkinson, R.S., *James Simpson and Chloroform*, London, Priory Press, 1973

Ballingall, Sir G., *Outlines of Military Surgery*, 4th edn, Edinburgh, Adam and Charles Black, 1852

Barling, S. and Morrison, J.T., *A Manual of War Surgery*, London, Frowde and Hodder and Stoughton, 1919

Beal, E. (ed.), *The Trial of Adelaide Bartlett for Murder, complete and revised report*, London, Stevens and Haynes, 1886

Beaney, J.G., *History and Progress of Surgery*, F.F. Baillière, Melbourne, 1877

Bigelow, H.J., 'A History of the Discovery of Modern Anaesthesia', in *A Century of American Medicine*, Philadelphia, Henry C. Lee, 1876

——, 'Insensibility During Surgical Operations Produced by Inhalation', *Boston Med. Surg. J.*, 35, (1846), pp. 309–17

Bishop, W.J., *The Early History of Surgery*, London, Hale, 1960

Bolitho, H. (ed.), *Further Letters of Queen Victoria, From the Archives of the House of Brandenburg-Prussia*, tr. J. Pudney and Lord Sudley, London, Thornton Butterworth Ltd, 1938

Bosell, C. and Thompson, L., *The Girls in Nightmare House*, London, Gold Medal Books, 1959

Bridges, Y., *Poison and Adelaide Bartlett*, London, Hutchinson, 1962 and 1970

Brock, W.H., *Justus von Liebig the Chemical Gatekeeper*, Cambridge, Cambridge University Press, 1997

Buxton, D.W., *Anaesthetics and their Administration*, London, H.K. Lewis, 1888

Cartwright, F.F., *The English Pioneers of Anaesthesia*, Bristol, John Wright and Sons Ltd, 1952

Case, A., *Day by Day at Lucknow*, London, Richard Bentley, 1858

Channing, W., *A Treatise on Etherisation in Childbirth*, Boston, William D. Ticknor and Co., 1848

Clarke K., *The Pimlico Murder, the Strange Case of Adelaide Bartlett*, London, Souvenir, 1990

Cole, J.J., *Military Surgery, Being the Experience of Field Practice in India During the Years 1848 and 1849*, London, S. Highley & Sons, 1852, reprinted 1856

Cunningham, H.H., *Doctors in Grey, the Confederate Medical Service*, Louisiana, Louisiana State University Press, 1958

Crombie, J.M., *The Induction of Sleep and Insensibility to Pain by the Self-administration of Anaesthetics*, London, J. and A. Churchill, 1873

Dantes, A., *Dictionnaire Biographique et Bibliographique des Hommes les Plus Remarquables*, Paris, Aug. Boyer et Cie, 1875

Davy, H., *Researches, Chemical and Philosophical; Chiefly Concerning Nitrous Oxide*, London, J. Johnson, 1800

Dorsey, J.S., *Elements of Surgery*, 2 vols, Philadelphia, Edward Parker and Kimber & Conrad, 1813

Duncum, B., *The Development of Inhalation Anaesthesia*, London, Oxford University Press, 1947

Duns, J., *Sir James Young Simpson, Bart*, Edinburgh, Edmonston and Douglas, 1873

Edwardes M., *A Season In Hell*, London, Hamish Hamilton 1973

Ellis, R.H. (ed.), *The Casebooks of Dr John Snow*, London, Wellcome Institute for the History of Medicine, 1994

Ellmann, R., *Oscar Wilde*, Great Britain, Penguin, 1988

Emerson, E.W., *A History of the Gift of Painless Surgery*, Boston, Houghton Mifflin and Co., 1896

Encyclopaedia of Medical History, New York, McGraw Hill, 1985

Esdaile, J., *The Introduction of Mesmerism into the Public Hospitals of India*, London, W. Kent and Co., 1856

Farr, A.D., 'Religious Opposition to Obstetric Anaesthesia – a Myth?', *Annals of Science*, 40 (1983), pp. 159–77

Forrest, D.W. (ed.), *Letters of Dr John Brown*, London, Adam and Charles Black, 1907

Frerichs, R.R., *The John Snow Site*, Dept of Epidemiology, University of California, Los Angeles. www.ph.ucla.edu/epi/snow.html (accessed May 2003)

Friedland, M.L., *The Death of Old Man Rice*, New York, New York University Press, 1994

Fülöp-Miller, R., *Triumph over Pain*, New York, The Literary Guild of America Inc., 1938

Gardner, H.B., *The History of Surgical Anaesthesia*, London, Baillière Tindall and Cox, 1896

Gillett, M.C., *The Army Medical Department 1818–1865*, Washington, Center of Military History, United States Army, 1987

Glover, R.M., *The Physiological and Medicinal Properties of Bromine and its Compounds . . .*, Edinburgh, J. Stark, 1842

Godlee, R.J., *Lord Lister*, London, Macmillan, 1917

Gordon, H.L., *Sir James Young Simpson and Chloroform*, London, T. Fisher Unwin, 1897

Gream, G.T., *Remarks on the Employment of Anaesthetic Agents in Midwifery*, London, John Churchill, 1848

——, *The Misapplication of Anaesthesia in Childbirth Exemplified by Facts*, London, John Churchill, 1849

——, *The Retention of the Mental Functions during the Employment of Chloroform in Parturition*, London, John Churchill, 1853

Grieve, M., *A Modern Herbal*, Harmondsworth, Penguin 1977

Griffiths, A., *Mysteries of Police and Crime*, 3 vols, London, Cassell, 1902

Guthrie, G.J., *Commentaries on the Surgery of the War in Portugal, Spain, France and the Netherlands 1808–1815*, 5th edn, London, J. Churchill, 1853

——, *Commentaries on the Surgery of the War in Portugal, Spain, France and the Netherlands 1808–1815, with additions relating to those in the Crimea in 1854–5*, 6th edn, London, J. Churchill, 1855

Guthrie, O., *Memoirs of Dr Samuel Guthrie and the History of the Discovery of Chloroform*, Chicago, G.K. Hazlitt and Co., 1887

Guthrie, S., 'New Mode of Preparing a Spirituous Solution of Chloric Ether', *American Journal of Science*, vol. XXI, I, art. VI, pp. 64–5

Gwathmey, J.T., *Anesthesia*, London, J. and A. Churchill, 1925

Hancorn, J.R., *Observations on Chloroform in Parturition*, London, Smith Elder and Co., 1848

Hennen, J., *Principles of Military Surgery*, Edinburgh, Archibald Constable and Co., 1820

Hewitt, F.W., *Anaesthetics and their Administration*, London, Charles Griffin and Co., 1893
——, *Anaesthetics and their Administration*, 2nd edn, revised and enlarged, London, Macmillan and Co., 1912
——, *An Inquiry Concerning the Safety and Sphere of Applicability of Chloroform in Dental Surgery*, London, J. Bale and Sons, 1895
Hibbert, C. (ed.), *Lives and Letters. Queen Victoria in her Letters and Journals*, Harmondworth, Penguin, 1985
Inglis, J., *The Siege of Lucknow, a Diary by the Honourable Lady Inglis*, London, Osgood, 1892
International Agency for Research on Cancer, *Chloroform, IARC Summary and Evaluation*, vol. 1, International Agency for Research on Cancer, 1972
——, *Chloroform, IARC Summary and Evaluation*, vol. 20, International Agency for Research on Cancer, 1979
——, *Chloroform, IARC Summary and Evaluation, Supplement 7*, International Agency for Research on Cancer, 1987
Kaye, G., *Manual of Army Anaesthetic Apparatus*, Melbourne, Australian Military Forces, 1942
Kidd, C., *Chloroform and Substitutes for Relief in Pain*, London, Renshaw, 1872
——, *On Aether and Chloroform as Anaesthetics, being the Result of about 11,000 Administrations of These Agents, Personally Studied in the Hospitals of London, Paris, etc., during the Last Ten Years*, 2nd edn, London, Renshaw, 1858
Kihlstrom, J.F., *Hypnosis and Pain: Prelude to the Modern Era*, Plenary address presented at the annual meeting of the American Pain Society, Atlanta, Georgia, November 3, 2000
Kirk, R., *A New Theory of Chloroform Syncope, Showing how the Anaesthetic Ought to be Administered*, Glasgow, John Menzies and Co., 1890
Lawrie, E., *Chloroform, a Manual for Students and Practitioners*, London, J. and A. Churchill, 1901
——, Brunton, T.L., Bomford, G., and Hakim, R.D., *Report of the Hyderabad Chloroform Commission*, Bombay, The Times of India Steam Press, 1891
Levy, A.G., *Chloroform Anaesthesia*, London, John Bale Sons and Danielsson 1922
Lister, J., *The Collected Papers of Joseph, Baron Lister*, vol. 1(1), 'On Anaesthetics', Oxford, Clarendon Press, 1909
Lyman, H.M., *Artificial Anaesthesia and Anaesthetics*, New York, William Wood and Co., 1881

Macleod, G., *Notes on Surgery of the War of the Crimea with Remarks on the Treatment of Gunshot Wounds*, London, Churchill, 1858

Mann, R.D. (ed.), *The History of the Managament of Pain*, Carnforth, Lancs, The Parthenon Publishing Group, 1988

Masson, A.H.B., Wilson, J. and Hovell, B.C., 'Edward Lawrie of the Hyderabad Chloroform Commission', *Brit. J. Anaesth*, 41 (1969), pp. 1002–11

Medical College of Georgia, *Environmental Health and Safety Newsletter*, Medical College of Georgia, Fall 1999

Meigs, C.D., *Obstetrics, the Science and the Art*, Philadelphia, Henry C. Lea, 1867

Moreno, *Notes of Lectures of Sir James Y. Simpson* (1854), Archives of the Royal College of Physicians, Edinburgh

Morgan, J., *The Dangers of Chloroform and the Safety and Efficiency of Ether as an Agent in Securing the Avoidance of Pain in Surgical Operations*, London, Baillière Tindall and Cox, 1872

Nichols, T.L., *Esoteric Anthropology – The Mystery of Man*, London, Nichols and Co., 1875

Pakula, H., *An Uncommon Woman*, London, Weidenfeld and Nicholson 1996

Panel on Heath Services (papers), *Dispensing Error at Central Kowloon Health Centre*, Information Note, Kowloon, March 1998

Pawling, J.R., *Dr Samuel Guthrie, Discoverer of Chloroform*, Watertown, NY, Brewster Press, 1947

Pearson, E., 'The Firm of Patrick and Jones', reprinted in *The Mammoth Book of Murder and Science*, London, Constable and Robinson, 2000. Originally in *Five Murders*, The Crime Club, New York, 1928

Pétrequin, J.E., *L'Ethéisation et la chirurgie Lyonnaise*, Lyons, 1869

Plowden, A., *The Case of Eliza Armstrong*, London, BBC, 1974

Porter, R., *The Greatest Benefit to Mankind*, London, Fontana, 1999

Priestley, W.O. and Storer, H.R. (eds), *The Obstetric Memoirs and Contributions of James Y. Simpson*, 2 vols, Edinburgh, Adam and Charles Black, 1856

Richardson, B.W., 'The Life of John Snow', preface to Snow, J., *On Chloroform and Other Anaesthetics*, pp. i–xliv

Robinson, D., *A History of the Dakota or Sioux Indians*, Aberdeen, South Dakota, News Printing Co., 1904

Robinson, H. (ed.), *Anaesthetics and their Administration*, London, Henry Frowde, Hodder and Stoughton, 1920

Robinson, V., *Victory Over Pain*, London, Sigma Books, 1947

Schechter, H., *Depraved*, New York, Pocket Books, 1996

Shenstone, W.A., *Justus von Liebig, His Life and Work*, London, Cassell, 1895

Shepherd, J., *The Crimean Doctors*, 2 vols, Liverpool, Liverpool University Press, 1991

——, *Simpson and Syme of Edinburgh*, Edinburgh, E. and S. Livingstone, 1969, pp. 87–8

Silliman, B., '*Elements of Chemistry, in the Order of the Lectures Given in Yale College*, 2 vols, New Haven, H. Howe, 1830–1

Simpson, J.Y., *Answer to the Religious Objections Advanced Against the Employment of Anaesthetic Agents in Midwifery and Surgery*, Edinburgh, Sutherland and Knox, 1847

——, 'On a New Anaesthetic Agent, More Efficient than Sulphuric Ether', *Lancet* (1847:2), pp. 549–50

Simpson, W.G. (ed.), *The Works of Sir James Y. Simpson*, 3 vols, Edinburgh, Adam and Charles Black, 1871

Singer, P.C. (ed.), *Formation and Control of Disinfection By-products in Drinking Water*, Denver, American Water Works Association, 1999

Smith, G.W. and Judah, C. (eds), *Chronicles of the Gringos*, Mexico, University of Mexico Press, 1968

Snow, J., *On Chloroform and Other Anaesthetics*, London, John Churchill, 1858

——, *A Letter to the Right Honourable Lord Campbell Lord Chief Justice of the Court of Queen's Bench, on the Clause Respecting the Proposed Prevention of Offences Bill*, London, John Churchill, 1851

Squire, P., *Companion to the latest edition of the British Pharmacopoeia* 12th edn, London, J. and A. Churchill, 1880, p. 99

Stead, W.T., *The Truth About the Armstrong Case and the Salvation Army, being the Editor of the Pall Mall Gazette's Statement in Full*, London, The Salvation Army Book Stores, 1885

Sykes, W.S., *Essays on the First Hundred Years of Anaesthesia*, 3 vols, London, William Clowes (Beccles) Limited, 1982

Taylor, F.L., *Crawford Long and the Discovery of Ether Anaesthesia*, New York, Paul B. Hoeber, 1928

Tomes, J., *Dental Physiology and Surgery*, London, John W. Parker, 1848

Underwood, A.S., *Notes on Anaesthetics in Dental Surgery*, London, Claudius Ash and Sons Ltd, 1893

United Kingdom Department of Health, *British Pharmacopoeia*, London, The Stationery Office, 2001

United Nations Environment Programme, *Handbook for the Montreal Protocol on Substances that Deplete the Ozone Layer*, UNEP, Nairobi, 1993

United States Agency for Toxic Substances and Disease Registry,

Toxicological Profile for Chloroform, United States Public Health Service, August 1995 update

United States Army, Surgeon-General's Office, *The Medical and Surgical History of the War of the Rebellion*, 6 vols, Washington, Government Printing Office, 1870–1888

Velpeau, Alf. A.L.M., *New Elements of Operative Surgery*, ed. V. Mott MD, 2 vols, New York, Wood, 1847

Walkowitz, J.R., *Prostitution and Victorian Society*, Cambridge, Cambridge University Press, 1980

Waugh, B., *William T. Stead, a Life for the People*, London, H. Vickers, 1885

Whyte, F., *The Life of W.T. Stead*, 2 vols, London, Jonathan Cape, 1925

World Health Organisation, *Chloroform, International Programme on Chemical Safety, Environmental Health Criteria 163*, Geneva, WHO, 1994

Wright, A.J., *Gardner Quincy Colton's 1848 Visit to Mobile Alabama*, Paper presented to a meeting of the Anaesthesia History Association and the History of Anaesthesia Society, Bristol, 1999

Wylie, W.D. and Churchill-Davidson, H.C., *A Practice of Anaesthesia*, London, Lloyd-Luke (Medical Books) Ltd, 1966

Journals

American Journal of Science (Am. Jour. Sci.)

Anaesthesia

Der Anaesthesist (Anaesthetist)

Annales de Chimie et de Physique (Ann. Chim. Phys.)

Annals of Science (Ann. Sci.)

Archives Internationale de Pharmacodynamie et de Therapie (Arch. Int. Pharmacodyn. Ther.)

Archiv der Pharmazie (Archiv. Pharm.)

The Association Medical Journal (Assoc. Med. J.)

The Boston Medical and Surgical Journal (Boston Med. Surg. J.)

British Journal of Anaesthesia (Brit. J. Anesth.)

The British Journal of Dental Science (Brit. J. Dent. Sci.)

The British Medical Journal (BMJ)

Bulletin de la Societé de Chirurgie, Paris (Bull. Soc. Chirurgie Paris)

Clinical Anesthesia (Clin. Anesth.)

Comptes rendus de l'Académie des Sciences (Compte Rendus Acad. Sci.)

Edinburgh Medical and Surgical Journal (Edin. Med. Surg. J.)

The History of Anaesthesia: Proceedings of the Third International Symposium

Internationale Archiv fur Gewerbepathologie und Gewerbehygeine (Int. Arch. Gewerbepathol. Gewerbehyg.)

Journal of the American Institute of Hypnosis (J. Am. Inst. Hypnosis)
Journal of the American Medical Association (JAMA)
Journal of the British Pharmaceutical Society (J. Brit. Pharm. Soc.)
Journal de Pharmacie et de Chimie (J. Pharm. Chim.)
Journal of Physiology (J. Physiol.)
The Lancet (Lancet)
Liebigs Annalen (Liebigs Annalen)
The London Journal of Medicine (Lond. J. Med.)
Medical Chronicle (Montreal) (Med. Chron. Montreal)
Medical Journal of Malaysia (Med. J. Malays.)
Medical Times and Gazette (Med. Times Gaz.)
Medicine and Law (Med. Law)
Medico-Legal Journal (Med. Leg. J.)
Military Affairs (Mil. Aff.)
Monthly Journal of Medical Science (Monthly J. Med. Sci.)
New York Journal of Medicine and the Collateral Sciences (N. Y. J. Med. Coll. Sci.)
Pharmaceutical Journal and Transactions (Pharm. J. Trans.)
Pharmacy in History (Pharm. Hist.)
Physiology Reviews (Physiol. Reviews)
Postgraduate Medicine (Postgrad. Med.)
Proceedings of the American Philosophical Society (Proc. Amer. Phil. Soc.)
Proceedings of the Royal Society of Medicine (Proc. Roy. Soc. Med.)
Provincial Medical Surgical Journal (Prov. Med. Surg. J.)
Quarterly Journal of Science and Arts (Quart. J. Sc. Arts)
Risk Analysis (Risk Anal.)
Science
Scientific American (Sci. Am.)
Transactions of the New York Academy of Science (Trans. New York Acad. Sci.)
Union Médicale (Union Med.)
Virginia Military Institute Alumni Review
Water Research (Water Res.)
World Anaesthesia

Newspapers and periodicals

The Cambrian
The Concord Online Monitor
The County News and Chronicle
Environment and Climate News
The Illustrated London News

The Kendal Mercury and Northern Advertiser
The Liverpool Chronicle
The Manchester Guardian
The New York Times
The Northern Echo
Nursing Record
The Oxford University Herald
The Pall Mall Gazette
Poole and Bournemouth Herald
Punch
The Runcorn Guardian
The Scotsman
Sheffield Daily Telegraph
St James Chronicle
South London Observer Camberwell and Peckham Times
Sunday Times
The Telegraph
The Times
The Western Times

Archives

Adelaide Bartlett – minutes of Police Court proceedings, Public Record Office, Kew, ref CRIM1/23/7
Archives of Bellevue Hospital, New York
Edinburgh University Archives Special Collections
The Simpson Archives, Royal College of Surgeons, Edinburgh
Edinburgh City Archives
Records of the Colney Hatch Asylum, London Metropolitan Archives
Records of Births, Marriages and Deaths, and Census Returns, Family Record Centre, London

Regulations

US Food and Drug Administration (1976), *Chloroform as an Ingredient of Human Drug and Cosmetic Products*, Fed. Reg., 41:26842–5
United Kingdom, The Medicines (Chloroform Prohibition) Order 1979 (SI 1979 No. 382, amended by SI 1980/263)

INDEX